WISCONSIN PUBLICATIONS IN THE HISTORY OF SCIENCE AND MEDICINE

Number 2

General Editors

WILLIAM COLEMAN

DAVID C. LINDBERG

RONALD L. NUMBERS

1
Death is a Social Disease
Public Health & Political Economy in Early Industrial France
William Coleman

Ignaz Semmelweis

The Etiology, Concept, and Prophylaxis of Childbed Fever

Translated and Edited, with an Introduction,
by
K. Codell Carter

The University of Wisconsin Press

Published 1983

The University of Wisconsin Press
114 North Murray Street
Madison, Wisconsin 53715

The University of Wisconsin Press, Ltd.
1 Gower Street
London WC1E 6HA, England

First printing

Printed in the United States of America

For LC CIP information see the colophon

ISBN 0-299-09360-3 cloth; 0-299-09364-6 paper

Contents

Tables   vii

Preface   ix

Translator's Introduction   3

The Etiology, Concept, and Prophylaxis of Childbed Fever

Preface   61

CHAPTER 1   Autobiographical Introduction   63

CHAPTER 2   The Concept of Childbed Fever   114

CHAPTER 3   Etiology   120

CHAPTER 4   Endemic Causes of Childbed Fever   158

CHAPTER 5   Prophylaxis of Childbed Fever   163

CHAPTER 6   Reactions to My Teachings:
Correspondence and Published Opinions   168

Epilogue   250

Index   253

Tables

1 Mortality rates in the first and second maternity clinics of the Viennese maternity hospital, 1841–46   64

2 The effect of seasons on the incidence of childbed fever: monthly mortality rates at the Viennese maternity hospital, January–December, for various years   68

3 The effect of overcrowding on mortality rates: births and deaths in the first clinic, Viennese maternity hospital, January–December, 1841–1847   72

4 Mortality rates of the newborn at the first and second clinics, Viennese maternity hospital, 1841–46   78

5 Mortality rates in the first clinic, Viennese maternity hospital, January 1846–May 1847, after reduction in the number of physicians and examinations   85

6 Mortality rates in the first clinic, Viennese maternity hospital, after chlorine washings were instituted, June–December 1847   90

7 Mortality rates in the first clinic, Viennese maternity hospital, after chlorine washings were instituted, 1848   91

8 The effect of the study of pathological anatomy: mortality rates at the Viennese maternity hospital, 1784–1848   96

9 Mortality rates in the first and second clinics, Viennese maternity hospital, 1839–40, before and after male students were separated from female students   98

10 Mortality rates in the paid maternity ward, Viennese maternity hospital, 1839–48   124

11 Mortality rates in the first and second clinics, before male and female students were separated, 1833–40   131

12 Mortality rates in the first and second clinics, Viennese maternity hospital, after chlorine washings were instituted, 1847–58   131

13 Summary of mortality rates at the Viennese maternity hospital for crucial periods   132

14 Comparison of mortality rates at the Dublin and Viennese maternity hospitals, 1784–1849   142

Preface

Because of the drama and pathos of his life and work, many people have some idea of what Ignaz Semmelweis accomplished. Few have bothered to look further. Yet his great book, *Die Aetiologie, der Begriff, und die Prophylexis des Kindbettfiebers,* is surely among the most moving, persuasive, and revolutionary works in the history of science. Because it concerns birthing practices, it is also of particular current interest. Moreover, it contains, in one volume, the exposition of a scientific theory, an autobiographical account of the origin of the theory, and a good sample of the reaction of the scientific community to the promulgation of that theory. For these reasons, it seemed to me that a translation of the *Aetiologie* should be of general interest and that it would also be an ideal text for a course I regularly teach in the history and philosophy of science. My object in preparing this translation has been to promote awareness of Semmelweis's contribution and significance.

In 1941, Frank J. Murphy published an English translation of the *Aetiologie.* But Murphy himself later identified certain weaknesses in his work, and since the translation appeared in a journal, it was never readily accessible. But for all its weaknesses, Murphy's translation has done much to promote the study of Semmelweis's work, and it was certainly helpful to me in preparing this new translation.

The original edition of the *Aetiologie* is much better written than most scholars seem to believe; nevertheless, it is a book that profits from abridgment. I have abridged the text in three ways. First, I left out about fifty pages of tables. The remaining tables have been renumbered (the pages on which they appeared in the German edition are in brackets), and their contents are identified in the list of tables above. Second, I cut back significantly on Semmelweis's polemical and repetitious responses to his critics, which constitute the sixth chapter. Although I reduced this part of the book to about half its original length, Semmelweis's ar-

ix

gument should not suffer, since almost everything that was left out appears elsewhere in the book. I have usually provided, in brackets, a brief indication of the content of these longer omissions. Third, Semmelweis's sentences often contain redundant phrases; I have eliminated these throughout the entire text. Because I so frequently omit redundancies, I have used ellipses to indicate omissions only when one or more complete sentences have been omitted. Partly because of the abridging process and partly because many of Semmelweis's paragraphs consist of one long sentence, the paragraphs in this edition do not correspond to paragraphs in the original. As an aid to those who wish to refer to the German text, I have inserted, in brackets, page references to the German first edition at the beginning of the translation of the first German sentence from that page; these references indicate when one or more complete pages have been omitted.

Whenever possible I have inserted given names in brackets before surnames on the first occcasion that Semmelweis uses the surname unless, of course, Semmelweis himself provides the given names. I have also inserted, in brackets, abbreviated definitions of the technical medical terms that Semmelweis occasionally uses. The definitions are usually from the twenty-fifth edition of *Dorland's Medical Dictionary* and are given at the first occurrence of the technical term. Semmelweis frequently provides some bibliographical information for the books that he cites, but the information is usually included in the text and it is seldom complete. I have completed these references and moved them into footnotes. Since I contributed most of the footnotes, it seemed most practical to identify, with a bracketed comment, those footnotes that are substantially Semmelweis's. Unless there is such a comment, the footnote is my own. The German text has chapter titles for all but the first chapter, and the chapters are unnumbered. As an aid to the reader, I have numbered all the chapters and given a title to the first one.

In examining Semmelweis's figures, I found that some of the percentages do not derive exactly from the figures printed in the tables as their source. In many cases, this seems to have been because Semmelweis simply dropped final digits rather than rounding them off. Because it is impossible to determine the reason for the errors and because I want to present Semmelweis's figures as his nineteenth-century audience read them, I have left the figures as they appear in the German edition. In a few instances, however, where the divergence seems to be greatest, I have given what would appear to be the correct percentages, in brackets following the figures of the German text.

It remains only to thank several people and institutions who have generously helped me with this project. I would like to thank an understanding department chairman for a slight reduction in teaching load that provided time to finish the project, and Brigham Young University for a generous travel allowance that enabled me to do a lot of last minute checking of sources. I would like to thank the editors of *Medical History* for permission to use my essay on Semmelweis, which appeared in the pages of that periodical, as a basis for the introduction to this edition. In the course of preparing the translation I checked each of Semmelweis's quotations against the original source. In doing so I used the holdings of several libraries, especially the Lane Medical Library at Stanford University, the Eccles Medical Library at the University of Utah, the Library of the College of Physicians in Philadelphia, the Medical Library of Johns Hopkins University, and the National Library of Medicine in Washington. I very much appreciate having enjoyed access to these libraries and the help of their staffs. I would like especially to thank Dorothy Hanks of the History of Medicine section of the National Library of Medicine for help in locating and copying many of Semmelweis's sources. I would like to thank Randy Everett, Travis Tucker, Jan Chambers, Carol Metcalf, Lynn Stosich, and Vanesse Tracy for various kinds of help in preparing different versions of the text. I very much appreciate the help of Jim and Julie Siebach, who typed most of the final version of the translation. I also express appreciation to the readers and to the editorial staff of the University of Wisconsin Press for many helpful suggestions that significantly improved the quality of the final result. I must also thank my two sons, Christopher and Thaddeus, who were responsible for the wording of certain passages. Finally, I thank my wife, Barbara, for her unwavering confidence and encouragement and for her eagerness to turn every dull conversation to the lively topic of nineteenth-century Hungarian obstetrics.

The Etiology, Concept, and Prophylaxis
of Childbed Fever

Translator's Introduction

"My doctrines exist to rid maternity hospitals of their horror, to preserve the wife for her husband and the mother for her child." In these words, Ignaz Semmelweis summarized his own life's work. His career, however, came at a time when medical theory and practice were changing dramatically, and his work can therefore be viewed from several vantage points.

In the first place, he was among the earliest to adopt certain aseptic medical procedures such as washing with disinfectants and the use of nail brushes.[1] In this respect his work represents an important advance in practical medicine. Most of those who have written on Semmelweis have emphasized this aspect of his work, and there have been numerous discussions of the relative priority of Semmelweis and of Lister and Oliver Wendell Holmes, who adopted similar procedures at about the same time.[2]

Second, Semmelweis's work came at a time of significant improvement in the care of hospital patients. This was particularly true in the maternity wards with which he was associated. By the beginning of the nineteenth century, large gratis hospitals had been established in most of the major cities of Europe. These hospitals served two functions, both dictated by the humanitarian objectives of the Enlightenment: they provided both free medical care for the indigent and a virtually unlimited supply of disposable bodies, living and dead, on which medical students could learn and practice their crafts. Associated with these hospitals were special maternity clinics. Each year thousands of poor women, usually unmarried, went to the clinics to deliver. In ex-

---

1. Semmelweis may have been the first to insist on use of the nail brush in cleaning the hands before examinations and surgery. This is briefly discussed in György Gortvay and Imre Zoltán, *Semmelweis: His Life and Work* (Budapest: Akadémiai Kiadó, 1968), pp. 210f.

2. For references, see Frank J. Murphy, "Ignaz Philipp Semmelweis (1818–65): An Annotated Bibliography," *Bulletin of the History of Medicine* 20 (1946), 653–707: 688–707.

change for free medical care and for the services of the associated foundlings homes, these women submitted themselves for use as teaching specimens in the training of obstetricians and mid-wives. But the maternity clinics were dreaded by the very women they ostensibly served; conditions in the clinics were often hor-rible. Semmelweis relates that in one major Parisian hospital in 1786, as many as three patients were obliged to sleep in each four-foot-wide bed.[3] He also mentions that in Vienna, three hours after delivery, women were required to arise from the delivery bed and walk through a passageway to their own beds,[4] that women were sometimes obliged to use uncleaned linen that was still stained with the blood and lochial discharge of earlier pa-tients, and that the air of maternity wards sometimes reeked from the emanations of nearby dissection rooms.[5] But the clinics were especially dreaded because of their frightful mortality rate; often between ten and thirty percent of those who were admitted did not escape with their lives. They died, shortly after delivery, from a disease known as childbed fever or puerperal fever. Dur-ing most of his career, Semmelweis was associated with mater-nity clinics in Vienna and Budapest. His autobiographical ac-count contains graphic and moving descriptions of conditions in these clinics. Semmelweis himself was active in the movement to improve the conditions of patients;[6] he adopted measures to make delivery easier and more comfortable;[7] and, most impor-tant, he drastically reduced the incidence of childbed fever. Be-cause his work was associated with the improvement of the ma-ternity hospitals, he is usually mentioned in social histories of childbirth.[8]

3. See below, p. 153; German edition, p. 204.

4. See below, p. 74; German edition, p. 36.

5. See below, p. 113; German edition, p. 99.

6. He wrote petitions to the government in the effort to secure better facilities for patients. For example, see below pp. 108–10; German edition, pp. 85–98.

7. Lajos Markusovszky, Semmelweis's close friend and associate, recorded that Semmelweis had newly delivered patients carried back to their beds so that they would not be obliged to walk. Gortvay and Zoltán, op. cit., note 1 above, p. 48.

8. For example, see Richard W. Wertz and Dorothy C. Wertz, *Lying-in: A History of Childbirth in America* (New York: Free Press, 1977), pp. 45, 94.

Third, Semmelweis's work came just at a time when medicine was becoming emancipated from certain presuppositions about sexuality. In the early nineteenth century, many medical beliefs and practices were based on discrimination by sex. It is well known that women were systematically excluded from the medical profession, even from the traditional practice of midwifery. "By the mid-nineteenth century this process was so complete and so deeply institutionalized in society that it was necessary to rediscover the fact that women had been engaged in the healing arts in earlier times."[9] But sexuality was the basis of more subtle forms of discrimination as well. For one thing, the use of such standard therapeutic procedures as bloodletting seems to have been based in part on presuppositions about sexual roles.[10] Moreover, there was a particular range of disorders, such as leukorrhea, hysteria, and puerperal fever, that were specifically identified as women's diseases.[11] Through the second half of the century, however, these forms of sexual bias were reduced or eliminated. Women were gradually admitted to the medical profession. There was a revolution in therapeutics that virtually eliminated many of the earlier procedures which had been used to reaffirm and to enforce social and sexual norms.[12] With the adoption of germ theory, such diseases as leukorrhea and puerperal fever could be seen as simple infections that had no essential sexual significance. Germ theory, and the new prophylactic and therapeutic measures that were based on it, rested in part on

9. Noel Parry and José Parry, *The Rise of the Medical Profession* (London: Croom Helm, 1976), p. 164.

10. K. Codell Carter, "On the Decline of Bloodletting in Nineteenth-Century Medicine," *The Journal of Psychoanalytic Anthropology* 5(1982), 219–34.

11. Some of these diseases are discussed by Edward Shorter, "Women's Diseases before 1900," in Mel Albin, ed., *New Directions in Psychohistory* (Lexington, Mass.: Lexington Books, 1980), pp. 183–208. By the middle of the century it had already been recognized that men occasionally contracted hysteria, but it was still regarded as a predominantly female disease. K. Codell Carter, "Germ Theory, Hysteria, and Freud's Early Work in Psychopathology," *Medical History* 24 (1980), 259–74: 265n.

12. Charles E. Rosenberg, "The Therapeutic Revolution," in Morris J. Vogel and Charles E. Rosenberg, eds., *The Therapeutic Revolution: Essays in the Social History of American Medicine* (Philadelphia: University of Pennsylvania Press, 1979), and Carter, op. cit., note 10 above.

a new strategy for characterizing diseases. Semmelweis was among the first to use this strategy.[13] In this respect it is significant that the first step in Semmelweis's work on puerperal fever, like Freud's first step in his work on hysteria, was recognizing that either sex was vulnerable to a particular disease that had previously been believed to affect only women.[14] Incidentally, Semmelweis's own attitude toward women in the medical profession can be inferred from his comments that all the midwives he trained were more enlightened about childbed fever than Rudolf Virchow, the most famous pathologist of the time, and were better prepared to avoid it than the members of the Obstetrical Society in Berlin.[15] Thus Semmelweis's work reflects the changing sexual orientation of medicine, and it can, therefore, be viewed in relation to the development of modern conceptions of sexuality.

Semmelweis can also be viewed as a contributor to the theoretical basis of medicine. As we will see, Semmelweis seems to have been among the first to adopt a particular strategy for characterizing diseases, a strategy that subsequently became central to medical theory. Yet, while his contributions to the practice of medicine have been generally recognized, this aspect of his work has been almost totally ignored. Moreover, most accounts of Semmelweis's life and work are discursive and superficial narratives that, like many earlier discussions of other figures and topics in medical history, are so "lacking in critical framework as to be of almost no use to succeeding scholars."[16] In reading

13. This strategy and the claim that Semmelweis was among the first to employ it will be justified in the fourth and fifth sections below.

14. Strictly speaking, by the time of Freud, hysteria was generally known to affect men as well as women. At first, Freud seems not to have realized that this was the case. In any event, the disease was still believed to be much commoner among women, and often to be caused by factors associated with women's sexual roles. See Carter, op. cit., note 11 above.

15. See below, pp. 232f.; German edition, p. 477. By contrast, according to Parry and Parry, the common view at this time was that "only a man could combine the necessary scientific and anatomical knowledge with physical strength and precision in the use of obstetric instruments which would allow him safely to practice midwifery." Parry and Parry, op. cit., note 9 above, p. 169.

16. Charles E. Rosenberg, "The Medical Profession, Medical Practice and the History of Medicine," in Edwin Clarke, ed., *Modern Methods in the History of Medicine* (London: Athlone Press, 1971), p. 27.

these accounts one frequently has the impression that the authors relied exclusively on common knowledge or on secondary sources, and that they gave little or no attention to Semmelweis's own writings.[17] Some writers have recognized that in adopting aseptic procedures, Semmelweis may have been more dependent on theoretical considerations than was, say, Holmes.[18] But no one has attempted to explicate those considerations or to determine their relation to the theoretical presuppositions of his contemporaries or successors. For this reason, the endless debates about the relative priority of Semmelweis, Lister, and Holmes, or about the relation of Semmelweis to his teachers in Vienna, simply could not lead to decisive conclusions. Moreover, Semmelweis's theoretical presuppositions provide important clues to understanding the social context of his work. Because physicians treat as well as describe and explain, medical theories are socially immanent in a way that the theories of physics or biology, for instance, are not. Consequently, one must expect that medical theory will intimately reflect and be reflected by the social role of the physician. As suggested above, for example, changes in medical theory often correlate with social changes in the practice of medicine or in the organization of the profession. More than in many sciences, therefore, one would expect medical theory and the social context of the practice of medicine each to provide useful clues about the other. For these reasons it may

17. Murphy pointed this out with respect to one of Semmelweis's early critics, op. cit., note 2 above, pp. 690, 694. Matters haven't improved much since. The most accessible modern edition of Semmelweis's main book, *Die Aetiologie, der Begriff, und die Prophylaxis des Kindbettfiebers*, has been a reprint of the German first edition and was published in 1966 by the Johnson Reprint Corporation in New York and London. This edition is preceded by an introductory essay by Alan Guttmacher, who probably never looked at the text—he claims, for example, that Semmelweis "mentions only one author, Hippocrates, by name" (p. xxvi), whereas in fact Semmelweis mentions nearly one hundred, most of whom are quoted extensively. Still more recently, Sherwin B. Nuland managed to write an "interpretation" of Semmelweis with only one quotation from the *Aetiologie*, and perhaps because "rendering the true sense of Semmelweis's labored German into effective English has proved inordinately difficult," that single quotation was taken from a secondary source. "The Enigma of Semmelweis—an Interpretation," *Journal of the History of Medicine and Allied Sciences* 20 (1979), 255–72: 267.

18. Gortvay and Zoltán, op. cit., note 1 above, pp. 211–13.

be useful to consider the particular theory of disease that Semmelweis adopted and that is presupposed in his writings.

We will begin by considering more carefully the disease on which Semmelweis focused his attention—childbed fever.

II

Childbed fever seems to have been known in antiquity, but the modern name dates from the seventeenth century;[19] by the late eighteenth and early nineteenth centuries, the disease reached horrible proportions. Early in the nineteenth century childbed fever was typically characterized symptomatically. In one essay it was defined as "that disease which is ushered in, from the second to the fourth day of confinement, by shivering, accompanied by acute pain, radiating from the region of the uterus, increased on pressure, and gradually extending all over the abdomen, with suppression of lochiae and milk, much accelerated pulse, furred tongue, great heat of skin, and that peculiar pain in the sinciput . . . short breathing, the knees drawn up, and great anxiety of countenance."[20] In harmony with the general program of pathological anatomy, there were numerous attempts to replace such symptomatic characterizations with more precise anatomical ones. The anatomical characterizations usually focused on morbid structural alterations in the uterus. This seemed reasonable, since the disease appeared to be closely associated with the birth process and since autopsies often disclosed morbid alterations in that organ. Such attempts were not particularly successful, however, because the disease left a variety of different and apparently unrelated lesions. According to the basic principles of pathological anatomy, this suggested that puerperal fever was not a single disease but rather a cluster of symptomatically similar diseases, each of which should be associated with a unique set of pathological alterations. Most physicians who wrote on puerperal fever in the early decades of the nineteenth century

19. Ibid., p. 41.
20. C. M. Miller, "On the Treatment of Puerperal Fever," *Lancet* 2 (1848): 262.

adopted some scheme for classifying different cases of the disease, depending on the specific anatomical lesions that were discovered in autopsy.[21] However, some physicians found these distinctions to be artificial, and, moreover, there were many cases of the disease in which autopsy disclosed no pathological remains whatsoever.[22] As a result there was considerable controversy about the ultimate nature of the disease and about the best means of characterizing it. Through the middle decades of the nineteenth century medical writers often stressed the difficulty of adequately characterizing puerperal fever.[23]

There were many different theories about the causes and nature of childbed fever; in particular there were major disputes about whether or not it was contagious. The British and most Americans were impressed by instances in which the disease seemed to have spread from one patient to another, and they

21. This was especially true on the continent. Eduard Martin wrote that the usual terms 'childbed fever' and 'puerperal fever' were "inappropriate for scientific discourse because they encompass very different pathological manifestations." "Über eine im Winter 1859–60 beobachtete Epidemie puerperaler Colpitis und Endometritis," *Monatsschrift für Geburtskunde und Frauenkrankheiten* 16 (1860), 161–76: 161. In place of these terms most physicians used 'puerperal processes' and had a scheme for classifying cases that focused on the specific anatomical lesions that were involved. See, for example, Eduard Lumpe, "Die Leistungen der neuesten Zeit in der Gynäkologie," *Zeitschrift der k. k. Gesellschaft der Ärzte zu Wien* 1 (1845), 341–71: 342; and Carl Braun, "Zur Lehre und Behandlung der Puerperalprocesse und ihrer Beziehungen zu einigen zymotischen Krankheiten," in Baptist Johann Chiari, Carl Braun, and Joseph Späth, *Klinik der Geburtshilfe und Gynäkologie* (Erlangen: Enke, 1855), p. 423. Both Lumpe and Braun cite several other authors who recommended a similar approach.

22. J. M. Waddy, "On Puerperal Fever," *Lancet* 2 (1845), 671f.: 671. James Young Simpson, "Some Notes on the Analogy between Puerperal Fever and Surgical Fever," *Monthly Journal of Medical Science* 11 (1850), 414–29: 419.

23. "There is almost no disease which varies more than puerperal fever does in different cases, in the intensity of its symptoms, and in the forms which they assume. . . . There is no disease to which it is so difficult to assign a set of pathognomonic phenomena." Ibid., pp. 425f. "There are major difficulties in giving a satisfactory definition of puerperal fever because in most special cases it is impossible to identify a common characteristic criterion for this disease." Franz Kiwisch von Rotterau, *Klinische Vorträge über specielle Pathologie und Therapie der Krankheiten des weiblichen Geschlechtes*, 4th ed. (Prague: J. G. Calve, 1854), vol. 1, p. 600.

concluded that it was often the result of contagion. Continental physicians, on the other hand, although sometimes admitting that the disease could occasionally be contagious, reported instances in which the disease did not spread as one would have expected of a contagious disease, and they generally emphasized other kinds of causation. We will consider each of these opinions in somewhat greater detail.

In 1843 Oliver Wendell Holmes published an essay entitled "The Contagiousness of Puerperal Fever"; in 1855 the essay was reprinted with an introductory note and with an appendix containing additional references and cases but with no change in the body of the text.[24] Holmes's main object was to show that "the disease known as puerperal fever is so far contagious as to be frequently carried from patient to patient by physicians and nurses."[25] Holmes's conclusion and most of the specific case histories on which the conclusion is based are from earlier British literature. Holmes himself admitted, both in the essay and again in the later introductory note, that the position he espoused was a majority view. "A few writers of authority can be found to profess a disbelief in contagion—and they are very few compared with those who think differently."[26] But Holmes felt that the existence of the minority justified the essay.

Holmes cited nearly twenty cases in which physicians examined or otherwise treated patients with puerperal fever, or in which they performed autopsies on persons who had died from puerperal fever and in which other patients subsequently contracted the disease. This suggested that the disease was spread from patient to patient and that the attending physician acted as the carrier. Hence, Holmes concluded that there must be some conta-

24. The essay appeared originally in the *New England Quarterly Journal of Medicine and Surgery* in 1843; it was reprinted in Holmes's collected *Medical Essays* (New York: Houghton, Mifflin, and Co., 1883), pp. 103–72.

25. Ibid., p. 131.

26. Ibid., p. 129. A year before the first publication of Holmes's essay, the editors of *Lancet* reported that in a discussion of puerperal fever at a meeting of the London Medical Society "the chief apparent circumstance is the diversity of opinion . . . as to the nature, . . . the symptoms and the treatment of the affection. . . . One fact only respecting the disease was generally admitted, namely, its unquestionable contagiousness." *Lancet* 1 (1842): 879.

gion that was generated by puerperal fever victims and that could be carried to other patients. At the end of this essay he warns obstetricians against taking "any active part in the postmortem examination of cases of puerperal fever" and that "on the occurrence of a single case of puerperal fever in his practice, the physician is bound to consider the next female he attends in labor . . . as in danger of being infected by him."[27] Holmes considers cases suggesting that puerperal fever can be produced "by an infection originating in the matter or effluvia of erysipelas."[28] But he finds the relation of puerperal fever to other continued fevers to be "remote and rarely obvious." Thus while he mentions very briefly reports that "puerperal fever has appeared to originate from a continued proximity to patients suffering with typhus," he adds that these cases are so relatively rare that they "hardly attract our notice in the midst of the gloomy facts by which they are surrounded."[29] Holmes never suggests that patients suffering from other diseases or corpses of persons who died from other diseases present any special danger to delivering women. Indeed, he observes that "the number of cases of serious consequences ensuing from the dissection of the bodies of those who had perished of puerperal fever is so vastly disproportioned to the relatively small number of autopsies made in this complaint as compared with typhus or pneumonia (from which last disease not one case of poisoning happened), and still more from all diseases put together, that the conclusion is irresistible that a most fearful morbid poison is often generated in the course of this disease."[30]

Holmes did not believe that exposure to the contagion was necessary in order for one to contract the disease—it could also come about in other ways. Each time Holmes states his main point precisely he says that the disease is sometimes (or frequently) carried from one patient to another.[31] "It is not pretended that the disease is always, or even, it may be, in the ma-

27. Holmes, op. cit., note 24 above, p. 168.
28. Ibid., p. 164.
29. Ibid., p. 165.
30. Ibid., p. 162.
31. Ibid., pp. 112, 129, 131.

jority of cases, carried about by attendants; only that it is so carried in certain cases."[32] Following the British, Holmes distinguished cases arising from infection from other cases that were epidemic or sporadic. "It is granted that the disease may be produced and variously modified by many causes besides contagion, and more especially by epidemic and endemic influences."[33] In the chronologically later introductory note, he writes that his theory "makes full allowance for other causes besides personal transmission, especially for epidemic influences."[34] In the literature of the times, epidemic influences were generally identified with atmospheric or terrestrial factors that could not be specified with any precision.[35] Since these factors could not be measured, the only criterion for deciding whether a given case of puerperal fever was epidemic was the frequency of similar cases in the surrounding area.[36] Sporadic cases were neither epidemic nor infectious; one discussion ascribed sporadic cases "to difficult labor; to inflammation of the uterus; to accumulation of noxious humours, set in motion by labour; to violent mental emotion, stimulants, and obstructed perspiration; to miasmata, admission of cold air to the body, and into the uterus; to hurried circulation; to suppression of lacteal secretion; diarrhea; liability to putrid contagion from changes in the humours

32. Ibid., p. 123.
33. Ibid., p. 133.
34. Ibid., p. 107.
35. For example, in Robley Dunglison, ed., *The Cyclopaedia of Practical Medicine* (Philadelphia: Lea and Blanchard, 1849), one finds the following comments: "There are presumable properties in the air, yet unknown save in their destructive effects" (1:674); febrile poisons may originate "in a peculiar unknown pestilential condition of the atmosphere . . . invisible and without taste or smell [known only by its] noxious effects on the animal body" (2:177); variations in febrile diseases "have been ascribed to the influence of some atmospheric or terrestrial agency, of which little or nothing is known except the effects it produces in the propagation and malignity of diseases" (2:181). Lumpe says similar things, op. cit., note 21 above, pp. 345–47.
36. Holmes, op. cit., note 24 above, p. 113. See also W. Tyler Smith, "Puerperal Fever," *Lancet* 2 (1856), 503–35: 503. Semmelweis discusses the confusion in the concept of epidemics and observes that this confusion was partially responsible for the failure to discover the cause of puerperal fever. See below, pp. 85f., 121; German edition, pp. 50f., 118.

during pregnancy; hasty separation of the placenta; binding the abdomen too tight; sedentary employment; stimulating or spare diet; [or to] fashionable dissipation."[37] In addition to contagion, epidemic influences, and the multitude of factors recognized as responsible for sporadic cases, Holmes also believed, as did most physicians who wrote on the disease, that puerperal fever could arise spontaneously.[38] Some physicians also ascribed cases of the disease to providence.[39]

In 1845, two years after the first publication of Holmes's essay, Eduard Lumpe, assistant at the first obstetrical clinic in Vienna, published an informed and carefully documented summary of current continental opinions about puerperal fever.[40] Lumpe discussed the difficulty of identifying consistent anatomical remains in terms of which the disease could be characterized. He confidently asserted that the disease was predominantly epidemic—"this is adequately proved by occasional increases and decreases in the number of cases without any change in those factors most commonly recognized as causes, by the simultaneous occurrence of cases, and by the similarity of the course of those cases that are simultaneous."[41] Lumpe felt that the disease usually attacked the uterus and that this could be the point of attack even if autopsy disclosed only minor changes in the uterus itself. According to Lumpe, maternity patients were particularly disposed to the disease because "lochial secretions, the purpose of which is

37. Waddy, op. cit., note 22 above, p. 671.
38. Holmes, op. cit., note 24 above, pp. 139f., cites with approval a long passage in which a Dr. Blundell observed that "this fever may occur spontaneously." To say officially that a disease occurred spontaneously did not mean that it occurred without causes but only that the causes eluded observation. One can find passages in which this distinction was not carefully maintained, however.
39. Holmes severely criticized Charles D. Meigs for ascribing certain cases of puerperal fever to providence. Holmes, ibid., pp. 103, 125. This view was certainly connected with the fact that most of those who delivered in maternity clinics were unmarried.
40. Lumpe, op. cit., note 21 above.
41. Ibid., pp. 342f. Eduard Caspar Jakob von Siebold used the same argument, on p. 343 of "Betrachtungen über das Kindbettfieber," *Monatsschrift für Geburtskunde und Frauenkrankheiten* 17 (1861), 335–57, 401–17; and 18 (1862), 19–39.

to remove waste matter, can be retained or absorbed. This induces decay of the blood. The absorption of harmful matter is much more likely following delivery, as the epithelium of the womb is discharged and regenerated and lacerated veins are present." [42] In addition to epidemic influences Lumpe identified the usual range of incidental causal factors. These included general deprivation, worry, shame, attempted abortion, fear of death, dietary disorders, exposure to cold, local miasmas, difficult delivery and especially damage to tissue because of the use of mechanical devices in delivery, and the retention and subsequent decomposition of the placenta. [43] Lumpe also mentioned the British view that the disease could be contagious, but he clearly regarded contagion as a minor consideration. [44] Other writers observed that on the continent, obstetricians simply had no experiences that confirmed the British belief in contagion. [45]

Because puerperal fever was ascribed to such a wide range of different causes, there was nothing resembling coherent unified strategies for preventing or for treating the disease. The English, of course, disinfected their hands and changed their clothing after contacting persons with the disease, [46] but they insisted that the disease did not always originate by contagion, and no one imagined that these prophylactic steps would prevent all cases of the disease. In the early nineteenth century, so-called antiphlogistic treatments constituted an important part of therapy. These measures included bloodletting, dietary restrictions, purgatives, lotions to cool the patient, etc. Puerperal fever, like most fevers, indicated an antiphlogistic regimen and most of those who wrote

42. Lumpe, op. cit., note 21 above, p. 345.

43. Ibid., pp. 345–49. Braun, op. cit., note 21 above, pp. 485–87, lists thirty different causes for the disease; Braun's list is discussed by Semmelweis, see below, pp. 246–49; German edition, pp. 530–35.

44. Lumpe, op. cit., note 21 above, p. 348.

45. Kiwisch says this in *Canstattische Jahresbericht über die Fortschritte in der Heilkunde im Jahre 1845*, vol. 3, *Specielle Pathologie und Therapie* (Erlangen: Ferdinand Enke, 1846), pp. 430f. Semmelweis quotes this; see below, pp. 219f.; German edition, pp. 430f.

46. Edward Blackmore also recommended that physicians not neglect to wash their hair and *teeth*. "Observations on the Nature, Origin, and Treatment of Puerperal Fever," *Medical Examiner* 8 (1845), 292–304: 297.

on the disease endorsed this strategy.[47] On the other hand, it was usually the privileged classes—those who ate too much and too richly, who worked too little and thought too much—who became plethoric and who required antiphlogistic treatment. The poor usually required supportive treatment, the very opposite to the antiphlogistic regimen. Some physicians felt that since the women who suffered puerperal fever were usually poor, supportive treatment was necessary. Thus contradictory therapies were recommended for puerperal fever, and the therapy that was selected in a particular case was usually justified by a consideration of factors unique to the individual patient in question.[48] Moreover, since supportive and antiphlogistic treatments were intended to compensate for opposite conditions, in theory it could happen that the disease was caused by the very measures used to treat it. Needless to say, there was considerable confusion and skepticism in discussions of therapies for puerperal fever; contemporary physicians frequently complained that there simply was no known therapy that was effective against the disease.[49]

Explanations were similarly defective. Lumpe called attention to various facts about the disease—he noted, for example, that it was particularly frequent in the winter, that (even though this

47. In 1848 C. M. Miller wrote that when he observed symptoms of puerperal fever he immediately ordered "eight or a dozen leeches to be scattered over the abdomen." Op. cit., note 20 above, p. 262. See also Edward William Murphy, "On Puerperal Fever," *Dublin Quarterly Journal of Medical Science* 24 (1857), 1–30: 5f.

48. See, for example, Robert Lee, "Fever, Puerperal," in Dunglison, op. cit., note 35 above, vol. 2, pp. 231–47, p. 231. Smith, op. cit., note 36 above, pp. 533f says the same thing. On the continent Kiwisch, op. cit., note 23 above, pp. 660–65, as well as Braun and others, made similar remarks.

49. "After much discussion everyone comes finally to the same depressing conclusion that an effective procedure for puerperal fever has yet to be discovered." Ferdinand Adolph Kehrer, "Zur Behandlung des Kindbettfiebers," *Monatsschrift für Geburtskunde und Frauenkrankheiten* 18 (1861), 209–23: 210. Siebold, following an earlier writer, remarks that "there is perhaps no disease process against which so many different, often totally contradictory, methods of treatment have been recommended as has been the case for childbed fever"; after trying every procedure that theory or experience could suggest, one ultimately concludes that "they must all be rejected as useless and ineffective." Siebold, op. cit., note 41 above, p. 19.

contradicted the literal meaning of the name of the disease) it could occur before birth, and that it was almost always associated with the maternity clinics. He also pointed out that the Viennese maternity hospital included two adjacent clinics that were alike in every respect, and that one of these clinics had a much higher mortality rate than the other.[50] The only explanation that he could give for these facts was that they reflected differences in atmospheric and miasmatic influences. On the other hand, he also admitted that nothing was known about these influences except the very facts they purportedly explained. There was no attempt to explain how fear, shame, worry, or the trauma of a difficult delivery could all account for the same disease that was otherwise ascribed to atmospheric influences. Thus there simply were no adequate explanations for many observed facts.

This was the situation when, in 1847, Ignaz Philipp Semmelweis was appointed assistant in the first clinic of the Viennese maternity hospital—the same clinic in which Lumpe had worked just a few months earlier.

III

Semmelweis was born in Taban, the oldest part of what is now Budapest, on 1 July 1818. He was the fifth of ten children of József and Terézia Müller Semmelweis; József was a successful grocer. The family spoke a dialect of German, but Ignaz also became fluent in Hungarian. Semmelweis began studying law at the University of Vienna in the autumn of 1837, but by the following year, for reasons that are no longer known, he had changed to medicine. He was awarded his doctorate degree in medicine in 1844. After failing to obtain an appointment in a clinic for internal medicine, Semmelweis decided to specialize in obstetrics. On 1 July 1846, his twenty-eighth birthday, Semmelweis became an assistant physician in the Viennese maternity hospi-

50. Lumpe says, "Whoever doubts the power of local miasmatic influences should try to find some other explanation for the fact that through several years . . . for every ten or twelve patients lost in the second clinic, the first clinic loses four to five times as many." Op. cit., note 21 above, p. 347.

tal. There he was immediately confronted by the horrible reality of childbed fever.

In the early decades of the nineteenth century the Viennese maternity hospital consisted of a private ward for women sufficiently affluent to pay their own medical costs, and two gratis clinics. Obstetricians were trained in the first clinic, midwives were trained in the second. For several years the incidence of puerperal fever in the first clinic averaged between three and five times that in the second. For this reason, women particularly dreaded the first clinic and tried desperately to avoid being admitted there. Various commissions investigated the high mortality in the first clinic and measures were proposed to reduce it; all the measures proved ineffective. The prevalence of the disease, together with the ineffectiveness of prophylactic measures, suggested that the disease was epidemic. Everyone agreed that there could be no defense against the harmful influences of the atmosphere.[51]

Shortly after being appointed as assistant in the first clinic Semmelweis seems to have begun looking for the cause or causes that could explain the difference in mortality rates. He recognized that the two clinics—located side by side and even sharing certain rooms—were necessarily subject to the same atmospheric influences. This fact convinced Semmelweis that the difference in mortality could not be due to atmospheric influences—in other words, that the disease was not epidemic. He then began a tenacious quest for endemic factors that could explain the difference in death rates. He decided that overcrowding, rough handling, specific medical procedures, inadequate ventilation, dietary irregularities, as well as particular physiological or psychological conditions of the patients, could not explain the incidence of puerperal fever, since all of these factors were either equally operative in both clinics or worse in the second clinic. Semmelweis gave particular attention to factors that

51. As Semmelweis himself observed, "there can be no defense against childbed fever that is due to atmospheric-cosmic-terrestrial influences. Advocates of the epidemic theory secure themselves behind this indefensibility; they thereby escape all responsibility for the devastations of the disease." See below, p. 121; German edition, p. 117.

were different in the two clinics. For example, he tells us that he discontinued supine deliveries in favor of deliveries from the lateral position simply because that was the practice in the second clinic. "I did not believe that the supine position was so detrimental that additional deaths could be attributed to its use. But in the second clinic deliveries were performed from a lateral position and the patients were healthier. Consequently, we also delivered from the lateral position, so that everything would be exactly as in the second clinic."[52] Of course, these measures were without effect. At this time Karl Rokitansky, who was director of the Institute for Pathological Anatomy and who ultimately became the most prominent pathological anatomist in Europe, assisted Semmelweis by allowing him to dissect all the female corpses from the hospital. Semmelweis was able only to confirm the confused findings of other anatomists, however; he found no clear indication of the causes of the disease.

As Semmelweis later told the story, the crucial event in his quest for the endemic cause of puerperal fever occurred in March 1847. Professor Jakob Kolletschka, who had been his friend and teacher, died from a minor injury incurred while dissecting a corpse. When Kolletschka's body was dissected, pathological remains were found that were similar to those obtained in dissections of women who died from puerperal fever.[53] Semmelweis had already concluded that the puerperal state was not a necessary condition for inception of the disease—he noted that women could contract the disease and even die from it during delivery or even during pregnancy.[54] He observed also that when women died of puerperal fever their own newborn infants, both male and female, sometimes died of a fever that left similar pathological remains. From this he concluded that the infants also died of puerperal fever. "To recognize these findings as the consequence of puerperal fever in the maternity patients but to deny that identical findings in the corpses of the newborn are the conse-

52. See below, p. 87; German edition, p. 52.

53. See below, pp. 87f.; German edition, p. 53.

54. See below, pp. 80, 117; German edition, pp. 43, 106. Lumpe made the same observation, op. cit., note 21 above, p. 343.

quence of the same disease is to reject pathological anatomy."[55] Similar reasoning forced Semmelweis to conclude that Kolletschka also died from the same disease. "Day and night I was haunted by the image of Kolletschka's disease and was forced to recognize, ever more decisively, that the disease from which Kolletschka died was identical to that from which so many maternity patients died."[56] Semmelweis now took a remarkable and decisive step: "I was forced to admit that if [Kolletschka's] disease was identical with the disease that killed so many maternity patients, then it must have originated from the same cause that brought it on in Kolletschka."[57] It is easy to overlook the profound originality of this argument. Even if they had admitted that Kolletschka and the maternity patients had died from the same disease, Semmelweis's contemporaries would not have admitted that the causes would have been the same. As we have

---

55. See below, p. 77; German edition, p. 40, cp. p. 43. In this passage Semmelweis notes that this conclusion forced him to recognize that the whole concept of childbed fever was wrong.

56. See below, p. 88; German edition, p. 53. Erna Lesky notes that Semmelweis's first account of the discovery was published eleven years after the event, "whereas Hebra's and Skoda's versions given in the very year of the discovery—1847—and subsequently in 1848 and 1849, make no mention of this outstanding heuristic importance of the Kolletschka case. Hence it is more than likely that in reviewing the events that led to his discovery, Semmelweis in 1858 exaggerated the significance of this case." *The Vienna Medical School of the Nineteenth Century* (Baltimore: Johns Hopkins University Press, 1976), p. 185. But Hebra and Skoda did not purport to give historical accounts; their only object was to present and to justify a scientific discovery. Semmelweis says explicitly that it was his intention to present historically the events leading to his discovery. See below, p. 61; German edition, p. iv. Moreover, the account of Semmelweis's lecture before the Viennese Society of Physicians on 15 May 1850 clearly reports Semmelweis as having said that he was led to his theory by the difference in mortality between the clinics *together with* the pathological similarities between childbed fever and pyemia in surgeons and anatomists. *Zeitschrift der k. k. Gesellschaft der Ärzte zu Wien* 6 (1850) 2:cxxxvii–cxl: cxxxvii f. This was certainly an allusion to Kolletschka that no one in Vienna could have missed. I see no reason to think that Kolletschka's death was any less important to the development of Semmelweis's thought than Semmelweis himself tells us it was. This is the view taken by József Antall; see, for example, *Pictures from the Past of the Healing Arts* (Budapest: Semmelweis Orvostörténeti Múzeum, Könyvtár és Levéltár, 1972), p. 78.

57. See below, p. 88; German edition, p. 54, cp. pp. 40, 273, 342.

seen, they accepted the possibility of a whole range of causes. By reasoning in this way, Semmelweis shows that he was assuming a new characterization of puerperal fever—one according to which it had only one possible cause. This will be examined more fully in the next section.

The cause of Kolletschka's disease was known; it was the introduction of decaying matter into his blood from the contaminated autopsy knife. Semmelweis realized that students and other persons associated with the clinic—particularly he himself—were conducting autopsies and then, after washing with ordinary soap and water or without washing at all, were examining the maternity patients. The smell of the examiners' hands convinced Semmelweis that washing in the ordinary fashion did not remove the decaying organic matter with which they had become contaminated in the dissections. The lacerations associated with the birth process provided access through which the decaying organic matter was introduced into the patients' blood systems. The result was the same as it had been in Kolletschka. Thus, Semmelweis quickly identified the contaminated hands of the examining physicians as the source of the decaying matter that spread the same disease among the patients. In the latter half of May 1847, Semmelweis began to require everyone associated with the clinic to wash in a chlorine solution before having physical contact with the patients. The mortality rate in the first clinic immediately fell to about the same level as in the second clinic.

It is possible that Semmelweis first concluded simply that the increased mortality in the first clinic was due to a cadaverous poison. In the next few weeks, however, this hypothesis proved to be too restricted.[58] Within a short time of adopting the chlorine washings, Semmelweis noted that there were still occasional outbreaks of childbed fever. Some of these were due to students who were inadequately conscientious in the use of chlorine, but

58. Semmelweis suggests that he started with the hypothesis that the disease was due to cadaverous poison (see below, pp. 92f.; German edition, pp. 59f.), and Franz Hektor Arneth, an associate of Semmelweis's, said so quite explicitly. "Note sur le moyen proposé et employé par M. Semmeliveis pour empêcher le développement des épidémies puerpérales dans l'hospice de la maternité de Vienne," *Annales d'Hygiène Publique et de Médecine Légale* 45 (1851), 281–90: 287.

he traced other outbreaks to infection from other sources—for example, to a reeking ulcer and to a discharging lesion. In this way Semmelweis broadened what may have been his original hypothesis—childbed fever was due not only to cadaverous poison but also to infection by decaying matter from any source.

A few physicians immediately recognized the practical significance of these results and notified their colleagues throughout Europe. Ferdinand Ritter von Hebra, editor of a major medical periodical and a leading dermatologist, announced the discovery in editorials in December 1847 and in April 1848.[59] Hebra claimed that the practical significance of Semmelweis's work was comparable to the significance of Jenner's use of cowpox inoculations. Over the next few months Semmelweis and his friends and colleagues sent letters to various obstetricians and to directors of obstetrical clinics; they announced Semmelweis's achievement and requested responses. C. H. G. Routh, who had been a student in the first clinic and who had returned to his home in England, wrote a lecture on Semmelweis's work. The lecture was delivered in November 1848; it was printed in a prominent medical journal and reviewed in several others.[60] Friedrich Wieger, another of Semmelweis's students, published a similar essay in Strasbourg.[61]

In January 1849 Josef Skoda proposed that the medical faculty

59. Ferdinand Hebra, "Höchst wichtige Erfahrungen über die Aetiologie der an Gebäranstalten epidemischen Puerperalfieber," *Zeitschrift der k. k. Gesellschaft der Ärzte zu Wien* 4 (1847), 1:242–44; and "Fortsetzung der Erfahrungen über die Aetiologie der in Gebäranstalten epidemischen Puerperalfieber," ibid., 5 (1848), 64f. Both editorials, as well as other early documents related to Semmelweis's work, are reprinted in Tiberius von Györy, *Semmelweis' gesammelte Werke* (Jena: Gustav Fischer, 1905).

60. Charles Henry Felix Routh, "On the Causes of the Endemic Puerperal Fever of Vienna," *Medico-chirurgical Transactions* 32 (1849), 27–40. The lecture was delivered by Edward William Murphy, since Routh was not a fellow of the Royal Medical and Surgical Society, the society to which the lecture was delivered. For a list of the reviews, as well as for bibliographic information about many of the early papers relating to Semmelweis, see Murphy, op. cit., note 2 above, p. 654f.

61. Friedrich Wieger, "Des moyens prophylactiques mis en usage au grand hôpital de Vienne contre l'apparition de la fièvre puerpérale," *Gazette médicale de Strasbourg* 9 (1849): 99–105.

of Vienna appoint a commission to investigate the practical applicability and the statistical foundations of Semmelweis's work.[62] Skoda was a brilliant professor of medicine who ultimately became one of the leading members of the Vienna medical school. At this time, however, he was among the younger members of the faculty and was struggling against the unsympathetic conservatism of the firmly entrenched senior members. Skoda's proposal was initially accepted unanimously by the medical faculty. When the commission was named, however, it did not include Johann Klein, head professor of obstetrics, chief of the obstetrical clinic, and Semmelweis's immediate superior. Klein withdrew his support for the proposal. To some extent Klein may have felt threatened by Semmelweis's work. Investigations by the prominent Austrian medical historian, Erna Lesky, however, have shown that broader issues were involved.[63] Klein's hostility seems not to have been directed against Semmelweis personally so much as against the younger faculty members in general who were engaged in a power struggle with Klein and his associates. Semmelweis became one focal point in this struggle. Klein interceded with higher administrative authorities, and Skoda's proposal was ultimately overturned. Two months later, in March 1849, Semmelweis was discharged from the first clinic. His attempts to secure an extension of his two-year period of service, supported by Skoda and Rokitansky but opposed by Klein, came to nothing.[64] During 1849 Semmelweis was denied other appointments that would have enabled him to remain in Vienna and to continue his work.

These months were not without hopeful signs, however. Carl Haller, provisional adjunct director of the Viennese General Hospital, published statistics that supported Semmelweis.[65] At

62. See below, p. 82; German edition, p. 46.
63. Erna Lesky, *Ignaz Philipp Semmelweis und die Wiener medizinische Schule* (Vienna: Hermann Böhlaus, 1964), pp. 11–54.
64. Ibid., pp. 35–51.
65. Haller's paper, which was originally delivered 23 February 1849, appeared as Ärztlicher Bericht über das k. k. allgemeine Krankenhaus in Wien und die damit vereinigten Anstalten," *Zeitschrift der k. k. Gesellschaft der Ärzte zu Wien* 5 (1849), 2:535–46: 536–38. The relevant passages are reprinted in Györy, op. cit.,

Skoda's suggestion, Semmelweis undertook animal experiments that provided some confirmation of his views.[66] In October 1849 Skoda delivered a lecture that was very supportive of the practical significance of Semmelweis's work.[67] In the following May Semmelweis himself gave a lecture on his discovery that was generally well received.[68] In the next year a former colleague from the second clinic, Franz Hektor Arneth, gave lectures in Paris and in London.[69] But by the fall of 1850 Semmelweis seems to have become discouraged at his prospects in Vienna. After the continued hostility of the older faculty members and further frustrations in attempting to secure an appointment, in October 1850 Semmelweis suddenly left Vienna and returned to Budapest. There have been many attempts to explain why Semmelweis abandoned his struggle in this way. The most plausible explanation, the one given by Semmelweis himself and by his friend and colleague Lajos Markusovszky, was that he was simply unable to endure further frustrations in Vienna.[70] In any case the move was associated with a dramatic change in his relations to

---

note 59 above, pp. 34f. Semmelweis discusses this report, see below, pp. 72f.; German edition, pp. 280–82.

66. See below, p. 105; German edition, pp. 76–81.

67. Josef Skoda, "Über die von Dr. Semmelweis entdeckte wahre Ursache der in der Wiener Gebäranstalt ungewöhnlich häufig vorkommenden Erkrankungen der Wöchnerinen und des Mittels zur Verminderung dieser Erkrankungen bis auf die gewöhnliche Zahl," *Zeitschrift der k. k. Gesellschaft der Ärzte zu Wien* 6 (1850), 1:107–17. The lecture was reprinted in Györy, op. cit., note 59 above, pp. 36–45. For bibliographic information regarding some of the reviews and reactions to Skoda's lecture, see Murphy, op. cit., note 2 above, p. 656.

68. The lecture itself was not published, but there were minutes from the lecture and from the following discussions. *Zeitschrift der k. k. Gesellschaft der Ärzte zu Wien* 6 (1850), II:cxxxvii–cxl, clxvi–clxix, and 7 (1851), I:iii–x. These are reprinted in Györy, op. cit., note 59 above, pp. 49–58. Eduard Lumpe also wrote a response. "Zur Theorie der Puerperalfieber," *Zeitschrift der k. k. Gesellschaft der Ärzte zu Wien* 6 (1850), 2:392–98.

69. Arneth, op. cit., note 58 above; and "Evidence of Puerperal Fever depending upon the Contagious Inoculation of Morbid Matter," *Monthly Journal of Medical Science* 12 (1851), 505–11.

70. See below, pp. 105f.; German edition, p. 81; and Gortvay and Zoltán, op. cit., note 1 above, pp. 70–73. Erna Lesky gives a different interpretation, op. cit., note 63 above, pp. 62–78.

his former advocates and friends. From that time on Skoda and Rokitansky withdrew much of their support for Semmelweis; apparently neither Skoda nor Rokitansky ever so much as mentioned Semmelweis in their lectures.[71]

Over the next several years Semmelweis remained silent on the matter of puerperal fever—as he himself tells us, he expected that the truth and the importance of his work would lead to its ultimate acceptance without further effort on his part.[72] This did not prove to be the case. Most of the responses to his work were unfavorable; his ideas were consistently misunderstood and misrepresented; and he seems not to have been taken seriously in Vienna or even in Budapest.[73] Finally, in 1858, Semmelweis ended a decade of silence with a flurry of publications. In 1858 he delivered a series of lectures before the Medical Society of Pest; these were published later in the same year in an Hungarian medical periodical.[74] In 1860 he published an essay explaining the difference between his views and those of the British.[75] In

---

71. Gortvay and Zoltán, op. cit., note 1 above, p. 72; Georg Silló-Seidl, "Unveröffentlichte und Neuentdeckte Semmelweis-Dokumente," *Orvostörténeti Közlemények* 26 (1978), 187–210: 209. Although, perhaps on the basis of the practical significance of Semmelweis's work, both Skoda and Rokitansky recommended Semmelweis when the time came to choose a replacement for Klein. Lesky, op. cit., note 63 above, pp. 83–93.

72. See below, p. 62; German edition, p. v.

73. Ede Flórián Birly, Professor of Obstetrics at the University of Pest, never accepted Semmelweis's teachings; he continued to believe that puerperal fever was due to uncleanliness of the bowel. Gortvay and Zoltán, op. cit., note 1 above, pp. 81f., 122. See below, p. 109; German edition, pp. 136f. In 1856 József Fleischer sent a notice to the *Wiener medizinische Wochenschrift* announcing Semmelweis's success at the clinic of the University of Pest; Leopold Wittelshöfer, who was the editor, remarked sarcastically that it was time people stopped being misled about the theory of chlorine washings. *Wiener medizinische Wochenschrift* 6 (1856), 536.

74. Ignaz Philipp Semmelweis, "A gyermekágyi láz kóroktana," *Orvosi hetilap* 2 (1858), 1–5, 17–21, 65–69, 81–84, 321–26, 337–42, 353–59. Translations of the lectures are reprinted in Györy, op. cit., note 59 above, pp. 61–83.

75. Ignaz Philipp Semmelweis, "A gyermekágyi láz fölötti véleménykülönbség köztem s az angol orvosok közt," *Orvosi hetilap* 4 (1860), 849–51, 873–76, 889–93, 913–15. A translation is reprinted in Györy, op. cit., note 59 above, pp. 83–94.

the same year his main work appeared, *Die Aetiologie, der Begriff, und die Prophylaxis des Kindbettfiebers.*[76] Unfortunately, everyone seems to have felt that they already knew as much about his opinions as they cared to know; apparently almost no one bothered to read his book.[77] Few have bothered to read his book since. What one finds there is a crucial conceptual innovation. Semmelweis's argument in the *Aetiologie* repudiates the notion that pathological anatomy is the ultimate foundation of medicine; in its place he employs a new strategy that was destined to become one of the defining characteristics of scientific medicine.

IV

Perhaps the easiest and most natural way to characterize any particular disease is in terms of specific changes in the human body. Thus, at the beginning of the nineteenth century, diseases were generally characterized in terms of abnormal signs and symptoms that were observable under ordinary clinical conditions. For example, one influential characterization of hydrophobia was a "complete horror of fluids reaching to such a degree, that their deglutition becomes almost impossible."[78] However, these characterizations were vague and it was sometimes impossible to identify reliably the disease from which a patient suffered or had died; for example, it was often impossible to distinguish between hydrophobia and tetanus. Through the

76. The *Aetiologie* was first published by C. A. Hartleben's Verlag in Pest, Vienna, and Leipzig, and bears the date of 1861. Gortvay and Zoltán indicate that the book actually appeared in October in 1860. Op. cit., note 1 above, p. 132. The only English edition to date was a literal translation by Frank P. Murphy that appeared in the periodical *Medical Classics* 5–8 (1941), 339–773. Murphy himself pointed out some of the defects in his translation. Op. cit., note 2 above, p. 706.

77. For example, when the book first appeared, the prominent Viennese obstetrician Joseph Späth dismissed it with the remark that Semmelweis's views had been known for fourteen years. Gortvay and Zoltán, op. cit., note 1 above, p. 141.

78. From a lecture in Paris by Gabriel Andral. The lecture was reprinted under the title "Perversions of Sensibility: Hydrophobia," in *Lancet* 1 (1832), 805–09: 806.

early decades of the nineteenth century there were intense efforts to provide more precise characterizations in terms of internal structural lesions. If each disease could be characterized in this way, then at least in autopsy it would be possible, in principle, to determine precisely the specific disease from which a person had died. The study of these internal changes—pathological anatomy—rose to prominence in France just at the beginning of the century, and through the next decades it dominated medical thought and research throughout Europe. The rise of pathological anatomy brought important changes; by emphasizing observation and the accumulation of facts, it provided the basis for a positivistic attack on the unrestrained speculative theories of earlier decades. For this reason it is customary to identify the rise of pathological anatomy as the beginning of scientific medicine.[79] However, pathological anatomy left much of medical theory and practice intact. In particular, pathological anatomy did not alter the basic strategy of characterizing diseases in terms of physical changes in the human body.

As long as diseases are characterized in terms of some physical state—whether in terms of clinical signs and symptoms or in terms of anatomical lesions—it is always possible, in principle, for different cases of one disease to have different causes. Nineteenth-century physicians found this situation entirely acceptable. In standard texts, virtually all diseases were ascribed to various different causes. For example, physicians recognized that hydrophobia—a horror of fluids—could be caused by certain fevers, by physical disorders in the throat, by emotional or psychological factors, as well as by the bites of rabid dogs.[80] Characterizations of diseases derived from pathological anatomy, while more precise than those based on the study of symptoms, still allowed for the possibility of a variety of different causes. Thus even late into the nineteenth century, after numerous attempts

79. To take radically different examples, Richard Harrison Shryock, *The Development of Modern Medicine*, reprinted from the 1936 edition (Madison: University of Wisconsin Press, 1979), pp. 151–55, and Michel Foucault, *The Birth of the Clinic* (New York: Pantheon Books, 1973), pp. 146, 197, both identify Xavier Bichat, the French pathological anatomist, as the founder of scientific medicine.

80. Andral, op. cit., note 78 above, p. 806.

to characterize hydrophobia in terms of morbid alterations, fear was still regularly regarded as a possible cause of the disease.[81]

Characterizing diseases so that each disease can have various unrelated causes results in serious practical and theoretical limitations, however. First, given such a characterization, it is practically impossible to generate effective techniques for controlling the disease. If a disease such as hydrophobia can be caused in different and essentially unrelated ways, then no single set of prophylactic or therapeutic measures can be relied on to be consistently effective. It is possible that the prevention or treatment of one class of cases of a disease may require procedures exactly opposite to those required in other cases of the same disease. Indeed, the very steps necessary to control one cause of a given disease could themselves constitute a different cause of that same disease.[82] This makes prevention and treatment so complex and confusing that effective practical medicine is all but impossible. Second, with these characterizations it is very difficult to generate simple and correct causal explanations for the observed facts. Through experience, one may accumulate a wide range of facts about any disease—for example, one may observe certain symptoms and find that these are regularly associated with specific anatomical lesions, that they have a certain course of development, that they spread to other persons in certain patterns, that

81. For example, in 1877 the editors of *Lancet* warned against diagnosing psychogenic or "mental" hydrophobia as true hydrophobia because "just as prophecy has often no small influence on its fulfillment, the diagnosis of hydrophobia conduces to its apparent verification." Thus, although the editors "doubt whether there are any authenticated instances in which a disease unquestionably emotional in its origin ran a rapid course to a speedy death," mistaken diagnoses *may* be self-fulfilling. To help prevent mistakes, the editors point out that whereas in true hydrophobia the convulsive spasms involve "the larynx as well as the pharynx, . . . in mental hydrophobia the spasm is pharyngeal only." The editors also express the expectation that "microscopical investigation may become of great importance as a test of the accuracy of the diagnosis in doubtful cases." *Lancet* 2 (1877), 399f.

82. For example, physicians frequently identified both excessive and inadequate diet as causes of the same disorder. It would be possible that the measures adopted to correct one of these factors could cause the disorder by bringing about the other factor.

they occur at certain times and places, and that certain people succumb while others do not. As long as each disease is characterized so that it can have various causes, it is very difficult to construct satisfactory causal explanations for most of the observed facts. For example, assuming that hydrophobia can be caused by fevers, contusions, fear, or dog bites, and that each of these factors can also cause other diseases, how can one possibly explain the relatively fixed course of development of the disease or patterns in its dissemination? Thus, admitting the possibility of a variety of different causes obstructs both the discovery of effective techniques for controlling disease and the development of explanations for the observed facts.

Typically these difficulties were overcome as follows. Beginning with a disease defined symptomatically or in terms of pathological modifications, specific conditions were identified that were causally necessary for many or most of the recognized cases of the disease. The disease was then given a new characterization in terms of that necessary condition. This, of course, entailed reclassifying many particular cases, since the new definition would include some cases with different symptoms (but the same cause), and it would exclude other cases with the same symptoms (but a different cause). These etiological characterizations had both practical and theoretical advantages. Since every case of the newly characterized disease had the same cause, it was possible to develop consistent and reliable techniques for preventing and treating the disease. Moreover, since every case of the disease now had a common necessary cause, it was possible to explain many of the observed facts in terms of that necessary cause. This new strategy first became prominent in work on the infectious diseases, where its application is obvious. But many specific developments in late-nineteenth-century medicine can be understood as applications of this basic strategy in various areas of medicine.[83]

Semmelweis probably began his work looking for the cause that could explain the difference in mortality between the two clinics. He quickly found it to be decaying cadaverous matter

83. Carter, op. cit., note 11 above.

that was conveyed to patients in various ways. He had shown that preventing the spread of this matter reduced the mortality level to that of the second clinic. He also knew that fifty years earlier, long before physicians in Vienna began to contaminate their hands by performing autopsies, about one percent of the patients died from puerperal fever. His chlorine washings had, therefore, achieved about the best results that he could reasonably expect; the first clinic was averaging about the same mortality rate as the second clinic (where students did not perform autopsies), and about the same rate as both clinics before the adoption of pathological anatomy. Semmelweis could simply have concluded that he had found the cause of the excess mortality in the first clinic and that the residual one percent of cases were due to one or more of the other recognized causes of the disease. This would have been completely compatible with the possibility that the so-called sporadic cases that continued to occur in both clinics were due to various other epidemic or endemic factors. It would, in other words, have been completely compatible with the recognized etiology of childbed fever. Semmelweis did not stop here, however; instead, he took a radical new step— one that he could not justify by any evidence, one that was rejected by almost every person (friend or foe) who responded to his work. Semmelweis insisted that, without exception, every case of childbed fever was due to the resorption of decaying organic matter through the damaged body surfaces. Semmelweis judged that the decaying matter was usually conveyed to patients from outside their bodies. He hypothesized that in about one percent of the patients, the decaying matter was not introduced from external sources but generated internally.[84]

It is not possible to be certain exactly when Semmelweis took this crucial step. He himself did not publicly discuss his results until 1850; with the possible exception of Friedrich Wieger's,[85]

---

84. See below, p. 116; German edition, p. 106.

85. Wieger was an eyewitness to Semmelweis's discovery. In his early paper he discussed decaying organic matter and discounted epidemic atmospheric influences. On the other hand, he did not assert that the disease is always due to decaying organic matter or that other factors are never causes. Op. cit., note 61 above. Moreover, it would be hard to reconcile some later comments by Wieger

none of the earlier discussions of Semmelweis's work suggest that he claimed to have identified a universal necessary cause for all cases of the disease. Hebra's announcements claimed only that most cases of puerperal fever in the Viennese hospital were due to cadaverous infection.[86] In his lecture in 1848, Routh said that his remarks applied "especially to Vienna, although it is believed that similar causes are brought into operation in other countries, and might as effectively be combated."[87] This was a far weaker claim than anything Semmelweis ever published on the subject. Semmelweis and his associates also sent letters to many leading obstetricians announcing his results. One of these letters, written by Heinrich Hermann Schwartz, was ultimately published in a Danish medical periodical; in this letter Schwartz did not imply that all cases of the disease are due to one cause.[88] Moreover, the few persons who responded to these letters seem not to have understood Semmelweis to be claiming that puerperal fever had a necessary cause. James Young Simpson observed that he saw no difference between Semmelweis and the British on this matter,[89] and Christian Bernard Tilanus, while claiming to agree with Semmelweis, continued to believe that many cases of puerperal fever were due to epidemic influences.[90] Skoda's lec-

---

and by his associates with the idea that every case of the disease is due to decaying matter. See below, pp. 126–28; German edition, pp. 132–34.

86. Hebra, op. cit., note 59 above.

87. Routh, op. cit., note 60 above, p. 27. Routh also says that puerperal fever, "like all other fevers, may be very much modified by epidemic influences" (p. 38). Semmelweis would not have agreed with this.

88. The letter was originally sent to Gustav Adolph Michaelis in Kiel. Michaelis forwarded the letter to Karl Edouard Marius Levy in Copenhagen. Levy published this letter together with a critical response. "De nyeste Forsög i Födselsstiftelsen i Wien til Oplysning om Barselfeberens Aetiologie," *Hospitals-Meddelelser* 1(1848), 199–211.

89. See below, pp. 74f.; German edition, pp. 282–84. As Semmelweis noted, Simpson gradually understood more perfectly what was at issue between himself and Semmelweis; in an essay published in 1850 Simpson refers to Semmelweis positively. Simpson, op. cit., note 22 above, p. 429. However, Simpson continued to believe that some cases of puerperal fever were epidemic and not due to the resorption of decaying animal matter. Ibid., p. 427, and "Medical News," *Monthly Journal of Medical Science* 13 (1851), 71–81: 72, 78.

90. See below, pp. 188–90; German edition, pp. 310–13.

ture in October 1849 does not once suggest that Semmelweis purported to have found a necessary cause for all cases of the disease—Skoda describes Semmelweis's work as an attempt to reduce mortality in the first clinic to the normal levels.[91] Indeed, one of the respondents to Semmelweis's subsequent lecture noted quite explicitly that nothing Skoda said precluded the possibility that many cases of the disease were due to the usual epidemic and endemic causes.[92] Franz Kiwisch von Rotterau of Würzburg and Wilhelm Friedrich Scanzoni and Bernhard Seyfert of the Prague maternity hospital responded to Skoda's lecture mainly by objecting that Skoda had said nothing new. Kiwisch pointed out that the British had long expressed similar views;[93] Scanzoni and Seyfert objected only to derogatory insinuations about the Prague hospital and to the suggestion that the excessive mortality in Prague was also due to cadaverous matter.[94] Because Semmelweis himself published nothing during these months, it is possible either that Semmelweis had not yet concluded that puerperal fever was always due to decaying matter or that, for whatever reason, his associates chose to state and to defend only

91. Skoda, op. cit., note 67 above.

92. Theodor Helm said, in fact, that neither Semmelweis himself nor Skoda in his earlier lecture had excluded the possibility of such other causes as difficult delivery and emotional disturbance, and he suggested that such causes might be responsible for the normal number of deaths while infection from cadaverous poison might cause the extraordinary number of deaths in maternity clinics. This is recorded in the minutes of the discussion of Semmelweis's lecture, op. cit., note 68 above, p. viii. As we will see, Semmelweis had not excluded these possibilities in the sense of having proved that they did not exist; but he had at least denied that there were such causes. Skoda did not even go that far.

93. Franz Kiwisch von Rotterau, "Einige Worte über die vom Prof. Skoda veröffentlichte Entdeckung des Dr. Semmelweis die Entstehung des Puerperalfiebers betreffend," *Zeitschrift der k. k. Gesellschaft der Ärzte zu Wien* 6 (1850), 2: 300–306: 301f.

94. Wilhelm Friedrich Scanzoni, "Über die von Dr. Semmelweis entdeckte, wahre Ursache der in der Wiener Gebäranstalt ungewöhnlich häufig vorkommenden Erkrankungen der Wöchnerinen und das Mittel zur Verminderung dieser Erkrankungen bis auf die gewöhnliche Zahl," and Bernhard Seyfert, "Ergänzende Bemerkungen zu dem vorstehenden Aufsatze." Both appear in *Vierteljahrschrift für die praktische Heilkunde* 26 Literarischer Anzeiger (1850), 2:25–33 and 34–36 respectively.

these weaker claims. There is no documentary evidence from the years before 1850 that Semmelweis or his associates believed that he had identified a universal necessary cause.

Semmelweis's May 1850 lecture was not published in full; we know it only from the secretary's minutes, and from the recorded responses of those who subsequently discussed the lecture.[95] These sources make it quite clear, however, that by May 1850 Semmelweis conceived of his results as applying to every case of puerperal fever.[96] Moreover, it is very clear from the writings of those who responded to Semmelweis after the 1850 lecture that he, in contrast to Skoda and Routh, was generally understood to have advanced this claim.

Eduard Lumpe, who had preceded Semmelweis as assistant in the first clinic and who knew essentially everything that Semmelweis used to support his claim, responded to Semmelweis's 1850 lecture as follows: "When one thinks how, since the first occurrence of puerperal fever epidemics, observers of all times have sought in vain for its causes and the means of preventing it, Semmelweis's theory takes on the appearance of the egg of Columbus. I was myself originally overjoyed as I heard the fortunate results of the chlorine washing; like everyone else, I too have had the misfortune to witness many blossoming young women fall before this devastating plague. However, during my two years as assistant in the first clinic, I observed incredible variations in the incidence of sicknesses and death. Because of this . . . any other possibility is more plausible than one common and constant cause."[97] After numerous criticisms of Semmelweis, Lumpe concludes: "If adoption of the washings makes it possible to avoid even the least significant of the many concur-

95. Op. cit., note 68 above.

96. Ibid., pp. cxxxvii–cxl; and cp. also the remarks of Heinrich Herzfelder, the head secretary who recorded the minutes: "Bericht über die Leistungen der k. k. Gesellschaft der Ärzte in Wien während des Jahres 1850," *Zeitschrift der k. k. Gesellschaft der Ärzte zu Wien* 8 (1851), vii, also quoted by Semmelweis, see below, p. 210; German edition, p. 398.

97. Lumpe, op. cit., note 68 above, pp. 392f.; also quoted by Semmelweis, see below, pp. 223f.; German edition, pp. 443, 445.

ring factors that cause puerperal fever, then their initial adoption
was a sufficiently large service. However, whether this is in fact
the case, only the future will be able to decide. In the meantime,
I believe we should wait and wash."[98] After the May 1850 lecture, Scanzoni no longer objected that Semmelweis had said
nothing new; instead he rejected Semmelweis's theory as false.
Scanzoni clearly admitted the possibility that puerperal fever could
originate in the way that Semmelweis discussed. Yet Scanzoni
rejected Semmelweis's views on the grounds that the disease was
primarily due to atmospheric or miasmatic influences and that it
could sometimes be caused by such other factors as emotional
trauma.[99] Hermann Lebert, Professor at Breslau, wrote: "It is
questionable whether those who have died of this disease can
have been directly inoculated by poison from corpses. Semmelweis has elevated this possibility into a system. In any case this
would be only one of many possibilities of conveyance."[100] Anton Hayne, a veterinarian who claimed priority for Semmelweis's discovery while at the same time rejecting it as false, noted
that animals frequently contract a disease corresponding to
childbed fever and that this is a consequence of dietary errors,
injuries, exposure to cold, and so forth. He wrote that in cases
where none of these factors can be identified "the disease can be
attributed only to a miasma or to a contagium."[101] Paul-Antoine
Dubois, whom Semmelweis identified as the foremost French
obstetrician, held that while one could not dispense with precautionary measures to guard against contagion, the contagious ele-
ment is neither as effective nor as pervasive as Semmelweis

98. Lumpe, op. cit., note 68 above, p. 398; also quoted by Semmelweis, see
below, p. 225; German edition, p. 454.

99. Wilhelm Friedrich Scanzoni, *Lehrbuch der Geburtshilfe*, 3rd ed. Auflage (Vienna: L. W. Seidel, 1855), vol. 3, p. 1,010; quoted by Semmelweis, see below,
p. 209; German edition, p. 396.

100. Hermann Lebert, *Handbuch der praktischen Medicin* (Tübingen: H. Laupp,
1859), vol. 2, pp. 759f.; quoted by Semmelweis, see below, p. 221; German
edition, p. 436.

101. Hayne's claim to priority is recorded in the minutes of the discussion of
Semmelweis's lecture, op. cit., note 68 above, p. v. His other remarks are quoted
by Semmelweis, op. cit., note 76 above, p. 442.

claimed, and that even before delivery, other factors predispose women to the disease.[102] Joseph Hermann Schmidt, Professor of Obstetrics in Berlin, approved of obstetrical students having ready access to morgues in which they could spend time while waiting for the labor process. He asked how Semmelweis's hypothesis could be reconciled with the observation that the disease occurs in relatively few normal deliveries. He then admitted that while the resorption of decaying matter may be "one path that leads to childbed fever, it is certainly not the only one."[103] D. Everkin of the Paderborn maternity clinic wrote: "I could not imagine that this circumstance is the universal cause, but I was led [by your communication] to avoid undertaking any procedures on maternity patients after examining corpses." He then warned Semmelweis that nowhere is one more frequently tempted with the *post hoc ergo propter hoc* fallacy than in medicine.[104] Carl Braun, Semmelweis's successor as assistant in the first clinic, identified thirty causes of childbed fever; the twenty-eighth of these was cadaverous infection. Others included conception and pregnancy, uremia, pressure exerted on adjacent organs by the shrinking uterus, emotional traumata, mistakes in diet, chilling, and epidemic influences. He too rejected Semmelweis for refusing to admit that these other factors were possible causes.[105] Everyone who responded critically to Semmelweis's 1850 lecture objected to his claim to have found the one necessary cause for all cases of the disease.

We have seen that neither Hebra, Skoda, Routh, nor Tilanus

102. Dubois's remarks are quoted by Semmelweis, ibid., p. 458.

103. Joseph Hermann Schmidt, "Die geburtshülfliche-klinischen Institute der königlichen Charité," *Annalen des charité-Krankenhauses zu Berlin* 1 (1850), 485–523: 501; also quoted by Semmelweis, see below, p. 227; German edition, p. 463.

104. These remarks are from a personal letter Semmelweis received from Everkin; the letter is quoted by Semmelweis, see below, p. 228; German edition, p. 467.

105. Braun's thirty causes appear in op. cit., note 21 above, p. 451, and in his *Lehrbuch der Geburtshülfe* (Vienna: Braumüller, 1857), p. 914. In the first of these, published in 1855, he mentions Semmelweis in connection with his discussion of cause number twenty-eight, cadaverous poisoning. In the later version, however, although he discusses the same cause in the same terms, all references to Semmelweis have been dropped.

seems to have recognized that Semmelweis was making this claim. Remarkably, one finds exactly the same circumstance in the writings of those who endorsed Semmelweis after the 1850 lecture. Justus Liebig included a favorable reference to Semmelweis in his *Chemical Letters*, and Semmelweis spoke of him as a supporter, but Liebig's passage concludes, "certainly other causes of childbed fever will be identified. However, no unprejudiced person can doubt that the one identified so insightfully by Dr. Semmelweis at the maternity hospital in Vienna is among the causes."[106] After 1850 Semmelweis was frequently mentioned favorably by British physicians, but none of them seem to have recognized that Semmelweis was claiming to have found one single cause for every case of the disease.[107] Semmelweis mentions especially Edward William Murphy as sympathetic to his views.[108] Murphy, who delivered Routh's first lecture on Semmelweis, did mention Semmelweis favorably, but he explicitly acknowledged a whole range of causal factors. Two pages before a reference to "the valuable observations of Dr. Semelweiss [sic] on this disease," Murphy notes that "in hospitals seduced women are always an easy sacrifice; but, even among the affluent, powerful secret causes of mental depression may act with as much force, and expose them to its influences."[109] Even Franz Hektor Arneth, who spoke on Semmelweis's behalf in the discussions of the May lecture and who did much to promulgate Semmelweis's view in France and in England, wrote nothing to imply that every case of childbed fever was due to one cause.[110] In 1861 Ferdinand Adolph Kehrer published a long discussion of childbed fever; he endorsed Semmelweis's prophylactic procedures and

106. Justus Liebig, *Chemische Briefe* (Heidelberg: C. F. Winke, 1851), p. 714; also quoted by Semmelweis, see below, p. 217; German edition, p. 422.

107. For example, Simpson, op. cit., note 22 above, p. 429; Holmes, op. cit., note 24 above, p. 170; Smith, op. cit., note 36 above, p. 504; and Murphy, op. cit., note 47 above, p. 21.

108. See below, p. 175; German edition, p. 285.

109. Murphy, op. cit., note 47 above, p. 19.

110. In the Paris lecture, Arneth said only that decaying organic matter caused the excessive mortality in the first clinic; in neither lecture did he suggest that all cases of the disease were due to this cause. Op. cit., note 58 above, p. 284f.; op. cit., note 69 above.

even commended his work on etiology, but Kehrer still acknowledged the existence of epidemic childbed fever and he warned physicians that overcrowded hospitals, humid weather, and a prevalence of typhoid-like diseases were especially to be feared.[111] One cannot avoid the impression that there was much more agreement between Semmelweis's critics and his supporters than between Semmelweis and his supporters. The crucial difference between his critics and his supporters was how seriously they took his claim that every case of childbed fever was caused by the resorption of decaying matter. Almost without exception,[112] no one believed that he had identified a necessary cause. His contemporaries either failed to see that he claimed to have identified such a cause—in which case they may have thought they agreed with him—or they saw that he made this claim and they rejected it. Perhaps this was the reason why at least two of his critics noted that in all the literature on puerperal fever there was nothing that supported the view Semmelweis was advancing.[113] Semmelweis denied this,[114] but in this respect it was certainly true.

In his publications of 1858 and 1860 Semmelweis's views are made fully explicit. In his lectures published in 1858 he asserted without equivocation that every case of childbed fever was due to the resorption of decaying matter.[115] His essay explaining the

111. Kehrer, op. cit., note 49 above, pp. 214–16.

112. The most likely possible exceptions are Friedrich Wieger, as mentioned above, and Lajos Markusovszky, who was a longtime friend and colleague of Semmelweis's. Markusovszky defended Semmelweis against various critics. See Gortvay and Zoltán, op. cit., note 1 above, pp. 137–39.

113. Braun, op. cit., note 105 above, p. 921; and H. Silberschmidt quoted in Semmelweis, op. cit., note 76 above, p. 407.

114. See below, p. 170; German edition, p. 275. In the Budapest lectures of 1858 Semmelweis seemed much less concerned to establish the existence of supporting literature than he was in his book. In his lectures he did not refer to Skoda, Hebra, or Haller. Moreover, in the book there are some differences in his treatment of critics. For example, Tilanus claimed in his letter to agree with Semmelweis, but he continued to acknowledge the operation of atmospheric influences as the primary factor in the disease. In his lectures, Semmelweis pointed out the difference in their opinions (Györy, op. cit., note 59 above, p. 68), but in the book he simply quoted Tilanus's letter without comment.

115. Ibid., pp. 70, 78.

difference between himself and the British ends with these comments: "The important difference between my opinion and the opinion of the English physicians consists in this: in every case, without a single exception, I assume only one cause, namely decaying matter, and am convinced of this. The English physicians, while believing that childbed fever can be caused by decaying matter, recognize in addition all the old epidemic and endemic causes that have been believed to play a role in the origin of the disease."[116] In the *Aetiologie* Semmelweis says quite explicitly that resorption of decaying matter is a necessary cause for puerperal fever: "In order for childbed fever to occur, it is a *conditio sine qua non* that decaying matter is introduced into the genitals."[117] He frequently asserts that every case of childbed fever, without a single exception, comes about in this way.[118] Semmelweis also distinguishes quite explicitly between the necessary cause that he had identified and the purportedly sufficient causes that his contemporaries were claiming to have identified. He cites a passage in which Joseph Hamernik specified three conditions that must be satisfied in identifying the cause of any disease: "Does this cause always have the same effect? As an experiment can one always bring about the disease in this way? In those cases in which the cause does not bring about the specified disease, can the same reason for failure always be identified?"[119] These criteria are all for causal sufficiency—not one of them is satisfied by a cause that is necessary but not sufficient. Semmelweis rejects the first criterion and gives this as his reason: "I have injected rabbits with decaying matter; some consequently died from pyemia and others did not. Could we deny that the decaying matter was the cause of pyemia in the rabbits that died, simply because the matter did not occasion pyemia in all the rabbits?"[120] In this passage he is using 'cause' in the sense of necessity. Sem-

116. Ibid., p. 94.
117. See below, p. 149; German edition, p. 196.
118. See below, for example, pp. 109, 114, 120, 141; German edition, pp. 87, 102, 114–16, 179.
119. Joseph Hamernik, *Die Cholera epidemica* (Prague: Calve, 1850), pp. 247f.; also quoted by Semmelweis, see below, p. 216; German edition, p. 418.
120. Ibid.

melweis claims to have fulfilled the second condition by his experiments with rabbits—he ignores Hamernik's stipulation that the disease is always produced in this way. Finally, while admitting that he has not satisfied the third condition, Semmelweis notes that "instead, my etiology of childbed fever satisfies another condition that Hamernik has not posed, but one that constitutes a condition for a true etiology. Namely, I have reduced the disease by making harmless that which I have identified as its cause."[121] This assertion is not totally unambiguous, but taken together with his repeated claims that every case of the disease comes from the resorption of decaying matter, Semmelweis seems clearly to be saying that in any true etiology one must identify that necessary condition whose prevention will eliminate the disease, just as by preventing the resorption of decaying matter Semmelweis himself eliminated childbed fever in all those cases where resorption could be prevented.

Having thus identified a necessary cause for childbed fever, Semmelweis gives a new etiological characterization of the disease; he defines it as "a resorption fever dependent on the resorption of decaying animal-organic matter."[122] He characterizes pyemia as "disintegration of the blood through decaying animal-organic matter."[123] Several important conclusions follow from these definitions. First, it follows that every case of childbed fever is a case of pyemia; in other words, puerperal fever is not a separate species of disease but only a variety of blood poisoning.[124] Second, it follows that there never had been and never could be a single case of epidemic childbed fever, since atmospheric conditions neither create decaying organic matter nor convey it to potential patients.[125] Finally, it follows that Kolletschka, the male and female infants, and the puerperae all died from the same disease, and this is true regardless of what pathological remains, if any, may be found in autopsy.

121. Ibid.
122. See below, p. 114; German edition, p. 102; cp. Györy, op. cit., note 59 above, p. 70.
123. See below, p. 117; German edition, p. 106.
124. Ibid.
125. See below, p. 120; German edition, p. 116.

Given this new definition of puerperal fever, it follows trivially that every case of the disease is due to infection by decaying organic matter; but how could this definition (or equivalently the claim that childbed fever has this necessary cause) be justified? There were two kinds of justification for this new approach: one practical, one theoretical. First, the new approach clarified and unified the practical measures that could be used against the disease. There may have been cases in which patients were so terrified at the prospect of delivering in the first clinic that they began to suffer from the symptoms of the very disease they dreaded. Given the earlier symptomatic characterizations of the disease, such patients truly had childbed fever. But preventing these cases would obviously require prophylactic measures quite different from those required to prevent the cases that Semmelweis was considering. By recharacterizing the disease as he did, Semmelweis made it possible to focus attention on cases involving one particular cause, cases that could therefore be prevented by avoiding that one cause. If patients died from something else, say fear, that was lamentable but not his immediate concern. The recharacterization thus made it possible for there to be consistently effective prophylactic measures that, at least in theory, could be used to prevent all but the residual one percent who, Semmelweis believed, would suffer from self-infection. Of course, precisely the same cases of disease could have been controlled by exactly the same measures even if the disease were still defined symptomatically. But as long as the disease was defined symptomatically, those same measures would not work on other cases of the same disease, and the ensuing confusion made it virtually impossible for any effective measures to be identified. The introduction of etiological characterizations was absolutely necessary for the development of systematic medical procedures.

Second, the new characterizations had enormous theoretical advantages, and it is obvious from Semmelweis's book that he found these advantages at least as compelling as the practical advantages. As Semmelweis himself certainly recognized, the strength of his characterization lay in its explanatory power. Semmelweis drew from his account explanations for dozens of facts that had been observed and recorded but never explained. To choose only a few examples, Semmelweis explained why infants never died from puerperal fever while their mothers remained healthy, why the mortality rates of infants changed in certain ways, why women who delivered on the way to the hospital or who delivered prematurely had a lower mortality rate, why the disease often appeared in particular patterns among patients, why the mortality rate was different in the two clinics and why it had changed in certain ways through history, why infections were rare during pregnancy or after delivery, why the disease appeared to be contagious, why it exhibited seasonal patterns, why the disease was concentrated in teaching hospitals, why some non-teaching hospitals had a much lower mortality rate than others, and why the disease appeared with different frequencies in different countries and in different historical periods.[126]

In this respect the difference between Semmelweis and the others who wrote on the disease, for example Holmes or Lumpe, is the difference between day and night. In their essays Holmes and Lumpe use their accounts of the disease to explain nothing beyond the very facts that suggested those accounts. Thus, while Holmes's account was associated with certain useful practices, neither Holmes's nor Lumpe's account had any real theoretical or scientific interest. By contrast, Semmelweis provides not merely practical advice for avoiding certain cases of puerperal fever, but a complete scientific theory.

V

By the time Semmelweis published the *Aetiologie* his ideas had been widely disseminated and discussed. One disadvantage in the late appearance of his book is that by the time it appeared, everyone had an opinion (usually erroneous) about what Semmelweis believed and few bothered to read the only complete and authoritative exposition of his theory. Semmelweis hoped

126. See below, pp. 99, 100, 101, 115f., 118, 122, 123, 125, 133; German edition, pp. 67, 69, 69f., 70, 104f., 108f., 109, 121f., 123, 125, 145, respectively.

that his book would help to convince his opponents. The book not only failed in this, but also seems not even to have enlightened those who claimed to agree wih him.[127] His reviewers responded to his opinions just as his earlier critics had done. In 1862 Carl S. F. Crede reviewed the *Aetiologie* in the *Monatsschrift für Geburtskunde*. According to Crede, Semmelweis calls everyone who disagrees with him an ignoramus and a murderer. The reviewer writes that Semmelweis's assertions "go too far and are too one-sided. In any case, Semmelweis owes us a proof that only the one etiological condition that he identifies is responsible. Nearly every obstetrician is still of the opinion that a large number of cases of illness remain that originate from a different cause, a cause admittedly yet unknown."[128] After what was obviously a more careful examination of the *Aetiologie*, August Breisky, an obstetrician in Prague, rejected Semmelweis's book as "naive" and he referred to it as "the Koran of puerperal theology."[129] Breisky objected that Semmelweis had not proved that puerperal fever and pyemia are identical, and he insisted that other factors beyond decaying organic matter certainly had to be included in the etiology of the disease.[130] From our point of view it is difficult to see how objections of this kind could still have been raised. In fact, Semmelweis's contemporaries were fully justified in their skepticism.

127. After publication of the *Aetiologie* a few people mentioned Semmelweis favorably, but none of them seem to have accepted his etiological theories. See, for example, Kehrer, op. cit., note 49 above, pp. 212–16, Siebold, op. cit., note 41 above, pp. 346f. The same held true for those who subsequently adopted Semmelweis's views. For example, August Hirsch claimed credit for rediscovering Semmelweis and for recognizing the significance of his work, but Hirsch explicitly denied that decaying organic matter was the only cause of childbed fever. *Handbuch der historisch-geographischen Pathologie* (Erlangen: Enke, 1862–64), vol. 2, pp. 423f. Semmelweis also received a few letters congratulating him on the publication of the *Aetiologie*. Toward the end of his life he published these letters as part of an open response to some of his critics. The letters mention only his practical prophylactic measures. Györy, op. cit., note 59 above, pp. 465–67.

128. Crede's review appeared in *Monatsschrift für Geburtskunde und Frauenkrankheiten* 18 (1862), 406f.: 407.

129. The review appeared in *Vierteljahrschrift für die praktische Heilkunde* 18 Literarischer Anzeiger (1861), 2:1–13. The remarks quoted above appear on p. 1.

130. Ibid., p. 12.

No doubt many factors contributed to the opposition Semmelweis continued to encounter. First, there was the continuing hostility of the senior faculty members in Vienna. This hostility may have been generated by political rather than substantive issues, but it remained real. Carl Braun, Semmelweis's successor in the first clinic, achieved fame and influence both in Vienna and in Budapest by submitting entirely to the unenlightened but orthodox opinions of Johann Klein.[131] Second, there was the fact that Semmelweis was consistently misunderstood and misrepresented. Hebra's first editorial suggested that Semmelweis believed himself to have discovered that cadaverous matter exerted harmful influences even through the uninjured skin of anatomists and surgeons. Routh and Skoda both described Semmelweis's discovery as concerning only cadaverous infection rather than infection from all decaying organic matter. Hebra, Routh, Skoda, and Arneth all suggested that Semmelweis's discovery applied only to the excess of mortality in the first clinic and to other cases that happened to be similar, rather than to every case of puerperal fever. It is possible that these misconceptions represent preliminary opinions that Semmelweis himself espoused in the course of formulating his ultimate views. In any case, by May 1850 Semmelweis held none of these positions; nevertheless his critics continued to argue as though he did. The ensuing confusion certainly retarded both the understanding and the acceptance of Semmelweis's views. Third, Semmelweis's discovery was subject to almost constant dispute regarding priority. The first foreign reaction to his work was a vitriolic letter from James Young Simpson of Edinburgh; Simpson complained that if Semmelweis were familiar with British medical literature he would know that the British had long regarded puerperal fever as contagious and preventable by precisely the methods that Semmelweis was claiming to have discovered.[132] When Semmelweis first reported his ideas in Vienna, a veterinarian claimed priority for the discovery.[133] Even modern expositors continue

---

131. Gortvay and Zoltán, op. cit., note 1 above, p. 162.
132. See below, p. 174; German edition, pp. 282f.
133. The veterinarian was Anton Hayne, see note 101 above.

to write as though there were questions about Semmelweis's priority.[134]

There were more serious obstacles that prevented acceptance of Semmelweis's doctrines, however. His most important critics understood his claims, and they were not distracted by questions of priority or by political disputes; their objections were more substantial. For one thing, given any of the accepted characterizations of puerperal fever, it was simply false that every case of the disease was due to decaying organic matter.[135] Everyone had known for years that the disease could be caused by cadaverous infection, but it was also obvious to everyone that many cases of the disease could not have originated in this way. Semmelweis's account would not have been plausible unless it included more than this. Unfortunately, almost all of his evidence related to infection from cadavers. His only basis for assuming that other kinds of decaying matter could also cause the disease was subsequent outbreaks of childbed fever that he attempted to trace to other sources of decaying matter. He noticed, for example, that during October and November 1848, when the mortality rate again increased dramatically, there had been two women in the wards of the first clinic who were suffering from reeking and discharging lesions.[136] He speculated that the increased mortality rate during those months was due to infection from these sources. But as his critics immediately recognized, there was virtually no evidence for this interpretation.[137] Remarkably enough, neither

134. Since the early decades of the twentieth century there have been interminable discussions concerning the relative priority of Semmelweis and Oliver Wendell Holmes; the discussions suffer from an acute lack of firsthand knowledge of Semmelweis's writings. For some of the earlier references see Murphy, op. cit., note 2 above, pp. 688–707.

135. As the disease was then characterized it certainly included (what would now be regarded as) a variety of inflammations and fevers, and probably did not have a necessary cause. See Smith, op. cit., note 36 above, p. 503; and Kiwisch, op. cit., note 23 above, pp. 600f.

136. See below, p. 93; German edition, pp. 59f.

137. Levy pointed this out in 1848 after first being notified of the discovery, op. cit., note 88 above, pp. 204–6; also quoted by Semmelweis, see below, pp. 181, 185; German edition, pp. 294, 301. Breisky developed the objection more fully, op. cit., note 129 above, pp. 6f.

of the women who supposedly infected the other women in the ward contracted puerperal fever. It seemed highly unlikely that a woman with a discharging lesion in her own uterus could have avoided childbed fever if her discharge was at the same time infecting the women around her.[138] These cases cast serious doubt on Semmelweis's hypothesis that decaying matter from persons who did not themselves have childbed fever could cause the disease in healthy persons, and also, therefore, on his claim that chlorine washing was responsible for the decline in mortality. As his critics pointed out, it seemed much more reasonable to ascribe the variations in mortality to changes in epidemic influences or in other unknown endemic factors. Since these cases were the only justification Semmelweis could give for believing in sources of decaying matter other than cadavers, his whole scheme must have seemed speculative and dubious. This may be the reason why even his closest associates continued to speak of cadaverous infection rather than accepting his notion that the disease could be caused by infection from other kinds of decaying organic matter.

There was another related defect in Semmelweis's argument. Even if one granted the possibility that the disease could arise through infection from these other sources, it was obvious to everyone that other cases of disease would still remain for which there simply was no infection from any outside source. In order to maintain his thesis that every case of the disease was due to infection by decaying matter, Semmelweis hypothesized that in these cases decaying matter was generated internally. While one could easily imagine that this might happen, for example in a difficult delivery, Semmelweis was unable to present the slightest empirical evidence of its actual occurrence. Indeed, he admitted that because of the inadequate and unsanitary conditions in which he was forced to work, it was not possible to collect any evidence about self-infection.[139] Thus the assumption that the disease could come about in this way was entirely gratuitous; it was neither more nor less justified than the equally gratuitous

138. Ibid., pp. 6f., 11.
139. See below, p. 118; German edition, pp. 109f.

assumption of other epidemic or endemic causal factors. There was certainly no basis for Semmelweis's further assumption that self-infection accounted for every case of childbed fever that was not caused by the introduction of decaying organic matter from external sources. To all appearances this assumption was simply a means of protecting his characterization of childbed fever from empirical counter evidence. In spite of his pages of tables, therefore, Semmelweis actually had remarkably little evidence for anything beyond the possibility of cadaverous infection—a possibility that nearly everyone accepted without question. Several of Semmelweis's critics recognized, more or less clearly, that his whole approach rested on changing the meaning of terms—on what must have appeared to be nothing more than a linguistic subterfuge. From their point of view, Lumpe and Karl Levy were exactly correct in objecting (respectively) that Semmelweis had created an egg of Columbus and that his argument rested as much on unstated a priori assumptions as on facts.[140] To them his whole approach seemed narrow-minded, wrong, and pointless. Moreover, by basing his conclusions on new definitions and on a priori assumptions, Semmelweis seemed to be reverting to the speculative theories of earlier decades that were so repugnant to Semmelweis's positivistic contemporaries. Semmelweis's critics objected that he was merely creating a new system in place of the older ones.[141]

Finally, Semmelweis's doctrine repudiated pathological anatomy—the very foundation of early nineteenth-century medicine. Semmelweis claimed that Kolletschka, the male and female infants, and the puerperae all died from the same disease. He supported this claim by observing that the pathological remains in all these cases were similar. Given the contemporary commitment to pathological anatomy, this was probably the only kind

140. Lumpe, op. cit., note 68 above, p. 392; also quoted by Semmelweis, see below, p. 223; German edition, p. 443. Levy, op. cit., note 88 above, p. 204; also quoted by Semmelweis, see below, p. 181; German edition, p. 293.

141. Lebert, op. cit., note 100 above, pp. 759f.; also quoted by Semmelweis, see below, p. 221; German edition, p. 436. Levy also suggests this, op. cit., note 88 above, p. 209; also quoted by Semmelweis, see below, p. 184; German edition, p. 301.

of argument that would have been persuasive, but because he argued in this way, it is easy to overlook the originality of this position. In fact, perhaps to make his position appear more acceptable, Semmelweis seems to minimize the differences between his findings and those of the pathological anatomists. For example, he pointed out that he was not the only one to observe that infants of either sex could contract puerperal fever;[142] but in this respect he was definitely in the minority—almost no one else spoke in this way. Moreover, while at least one British physician suggested that surgeons died from a disease that was similar to puerperal fever,[143] only Semmelweis maintained that the diseases were identical. Lumpe, like most pathological anatomists, found it incredible that the cases should even be referred to as similar.[144] Lumpe had good reason to feel this way; Semmelweis himself admitted that the pathological remains in Kolletschka and in the other surgeons were not identical to those in the maternity patients—the remains were, in fact, totally different in the genital area, in the one area where all efforts to characterize puerperal fever necessarily focused.[145] Indeed, all existing characterizations of childbed fever referred either to the puerperal state or to certain morbid alterations in the uterus (and

142. See below, p. 77; German edition, p. 40. The French called attention to infantile puerperal fever in 1855, and their discussions were reviewed in *Monatsschrift der Geburtshülfe* 7 (1856), 152f., and in the *Wiener medizinische Wochenschrift* 6(1856), Journal Review, no. 3, p. 22f. I have not been able to identify this claim in any publications before Semmelweis's work in 1847. This must at least raise the possibility that this recognition was not part of Semmelweis's original thinking.

143. The British sometimes claimed that puerperal fever caused (and could be caused by) a poison that could also cause (and be caused by) such other diseases as typhoid and erysipelas, and these, of course, affected males as well as females. See, for example, Robert Storres, "On the Contagious Effects of Puerperal Fever on the Male Subject," *Provincial Medical and Surgical Journal* 19 (1845), 289–94: 290. For a similar opinion, see below, p. 145; German edition, p. 188.

144. Lumpe, op. cit., note 21 above, p. 348. Lumpe cites an essay by Matthew Gibson to justify his claim that the British believed men could contract a disease similar to puerperal fever. In fact, Gibson's essay isn't about puerperal fever and he doesn't even mention the disease by name. "Epidemic Fever," *Lancet* 1 (1843): 330–34.

145. See below, pp. 77, 117; German edition, pp. 40, 107.

usually to both). These characterizations excluded infants and adult males by definition. Moreover, as we have seen, no clear patterns emerged in autopsies of victims of puerperal fever; some corpses revealed no morbid alterations whatsoever, and the alterations that were detected in others varied enormously from case to case. The pathological remains did not warrant classifying even all the cases of puerperal fever together, and the pathological anatomists did not do so.[146] To assimilate all these cases and then to include the infants and the anatomists as well was to go directly counter to the basic principles of pathological anatomy.[147]

By now it is obvious by which principle Semmelweis was guided in his reevaluation of the evidence. It is possible that in the context of discovering the necessary cause of childbed fever, Semmelweis first noted a similarity in the pathological remains, he then inferred that the diseases were identical, and he concluded that the puerperae died because of infection by decaying matter. In the context of expounding and justifying his theory as a whole, however, he reasoned in precisely the opposite direction. If he had still taken pathological anatomy as fundamental, he could never have concluded that Kolletschka, the infants, and the puerperae all died from the same disease because they had different pathological remains. Given his etiological definitions, however, these differences could be disregarded as irrelevant. By the time he wrote his book, Semmelweis knew that the diseases were the same because they had the same causes. Moreover, Semmelweis had good reason to have more confidence in his etiological characterizations than in pathological anatomy. First, pathological anatomy could not prevent childbed fever—in a sense it caused the disease. The etiological characterizations made it possible to prevent almost every case of the disease. Second, while pathological anatomy could explain almost nothing, the new characterizations seemed to explain everything; they even provided a criterion for deciding which pathological remains were significant and which were not.

146. See above, note 21.
147. Breisky pointed this out, op. cit., note 129 above, p. 11.

In the face of these very fundamental objections, however, Semmelweis's critics were simply unable to accept his extravagant claims about childbed fever. Thus while most of them seemed perfectly willing to experiment with the practical prophylactic measures that Semmelweis recommended, virtually everyone either ignored or rejected his basic theoretical innovations. The practical and theoretical advantages of the etiological approach to childbed fever were not yet sufficiently obvious to warrant abandoning an entire medical system. This could come about only when subsequent work made it clear that the same new approach yielded similar advantages when applied to a whole range of different diseases.

VI

Because Semmelweis's theoretical strategy was so crucial in his own work and because the same strategy was so important to the subsequent development of medicine, it is interesting to consider the possibility that he may have drawn the innovations in that strategy from the thinking of his professors in the Vienna medical school. In her excellent monograph *The Vienna Medical School in the Nineteenth Century* and in an independent essay, Erna Lesky claims that Semmelweis "absorbed Rokitansky's and Skoda's methods of reasoning and investigation in a synthesis which brought forth revolutionizing new results."[148] Thus Lesky believes that Semmelweis obtained new results from the methods he learned from his professors. There is no doubt that Semmelweis was profoundly influenced by what he learned in Vienna; for example, as Lesky observes, his unremitting use of *modus tollendo ponens* may well have come from Skoda. Semmelweis's extensive use of statistics was also characteristic of the Vienna School and may have been learned there. For other crucial and decisive aspects of his method the case is less clear, however. Lesky claims that the training Semmelweis rceived in pathological anatomy while working with Rokitansky enabled him to

---

148. Lesky, op. cit., note 56 above, p. 183; and "Semmelweis: Legende und Historie," *Deutsche medizinische Wochenschrift* 97 (1972), 627–32: 629.

recognize that the anatomical findings in the patients and their infants were identical with those in Kolletschka, and so to conclude that childbed fever, previously thought of as a unique disease, was merely a variety of pyemia.[149] But neither Rokitansky himself nor any of his other students or associates—including Lumpe, Johann Baptist Chiari, and Eduard Mikschik—recognized the findings as identical.[150] The French and the British, not the Viennese, stressed the similarity between the pathological remains in maternity patients and in infants and in victims of pyemia (respectively). Lumpe, who was also an assistant in the first clinic, expressed astonishment at the British idea that men could contract a disease similar to puerperal fever.[151] Moreover, as we have seen, recognizing the similarity of the pathological remains required a reevaluation of the evidence and, to some extent, a repudiation of the basic principles of pathological anatomy. It is surely misleading to ascribe this aspect of Semmelweis's thought simply to his training in Vienna.

Lesky also claims that the Vienna school "provided Semmelweis with the intellectual tools to infer a single unified cause from identical anatomical remains."[152] This claim obviously relates more directly to what I have identified as a crucial step in Semmelweis's thought. Unfortunately, Lesky provides no support for this claim; she goes on immediately to point out that Semmelweis learned from Skoda the so-called method of exclusion, and that in seeking the cause of the difference in mortality between the clinics, he took this procedure out of its original symptomatic-diagnostic context and applied it in a new and original way.[153] It seems very possible that Semmelweis's systematic exclusion of one possible endemic cause after another was an application of Skoda's method; but that is something quite different from the quest for a necessary cause common to all cases of an illness. Semmelweis seems to have been among the first to conceive of puerperal fever in a way such that it would

149. Ibid.
150. Lesky, op. cit., note 56 above, p. 185.
151. Lumpe, op. cit., note 21 above, p. 348.
152. Lesky, op. cit., note 148 above, p. 629.
153. Ibid.

have a necessary cause—all of his contemporaries seem to have been thinking in altogether different ways. It would be useful to know whether Skoda ever unambiguously asserted of any disease that it must have a necessary cause; he certainly did not make such an assertion for puerperal fever. In his first lecture announcing Semmelweis's results, he said that Semmelweis had discovered the cause of the unusually high incidence of the disease among the patients in the first clinic and the means of reducing this to the usual number. He also noted that the difference in mortality between the clinics precluded any thought that the generation of the sickness was the direct operation of an epidemic cause, and he concluded that, common opinion notwithstanding, the high incidence of disease in the maternity clinic could not be thought of as an epidemic.[154] These assertions did not preclude the possibility that various causal factors were responsible for the usual incidence of puerperal fever or that epidemic puerperal fever sometimes occurred. As we have seen, Theodor Helm, who heard Skoda's lecture, pointed out in a later discussion that nothing Skoda said excluded the possibility that such factors as difficult delivery or emotional trauma could also cause puerperal fever.[155] In the years immediately after Semmelweis's work, Skoda wrote official documents on Semmelweis's behalf. In these documents he is consistently ambiguous in describing Semmelweis's views; he consistently speaks of the causes (plural) of childbed fever, and he never describes Semmelweis's work as a quest for the one necessary cause.[156] By contrast, during the same period Johann Klein, who rejected Semmelweis's opinions, consistently described Semmelweis's work as a quest for the cause (singular) of childbed fever.[157] There is also the

154. Györy, op. cit., note 59 above, p. 36.

155. See above, note 92.

156. Lesky, op. cit., note 63 above, pp. 21, 26. One of these documents explicitly asserts that Semmelweis was "not seeking to explain all the causes of puerperal fever, but only to find and to circumvent the causes of the excessive mortality in the first clinic." (p. 27).

157. Ibid., pp. 29, 43, 46. The contrast between Skoda and Klein may have been like the contrast between Semmelweis's other supporters and critics—the former did not take seriously his claim to have discovered a universal necessary cause, the latter admitted that he made this claim but rejected it.

interesting fact that long after Semmelweis had rejected the idea
that corpses were the only source of decaying matter which could
cause puerperal fever, Skoda continued to speak only of cadaverous poisoning.[158] Finally, we must recall that Skoda did not
speak in Semmelweis's behalf in the discussions of Semmelweis's
May 1850 lecture—the lecture in which Semmelweis first un-
equivocally claimed to have found the one necessary cause for
puerperal fever. Skoda's silence can be interpreted in different
ways; one possibility is that he was simply unable to accept this
aspect of Semmelweis's work but, perhaps because of personal
loyalty to Semmelweis, preferred not to make his disagreement
explicit. Even in lectures on puerperal diseases given much later,
Skoda did not assert that all cases of puerperal fever could be
ascribed to a single, necessary cause.[159] Of course, we know that
Skoda accepted Semmelweis's discovery that the high incidence
of childbed fever in the first clinic was caused by the unclean
hands of the medical staff and that chlorine washings could reduce the incidence of disease to the "normal" level. But there is
no clear evidence that Skoda ever understood, agreed with, or
shared Semmelweis's interest in a single necessary cause for all
cases of the disease, or Semmelweis's strategy of recharacterizing
the disease in terms of such a cause. Since this particular strategy
was the crucial step in Semmelweis's work, his achievement certainly cannot be thought of simply as a new application of Rokitansky's and Skoda's methods of reasoning. Lesky and others
have claimed that Skoda and Rokitansky were the "intellectual
fathers of [Semmelweis's] discovery."[160] In fact Skoda and

158. Thus in his lecture given in 1849 Skoda spoke only of cadaverous poison,
op. cit., note 67 above, while Hebra's announcement made two years earlier, op.
cit., note 59 above, Schwartz's 1847 letter to Michaelis, op. cit., note 88 above,
and even Wieger's 1849 essay, op. cit., note 61 above, all assert quite clearly that
other sources of decaying matter were involved. This cannot have been a simple
oversight on Skoda's part.

159. Josef Skoda, "Über Krankheiten bei Puerpern," *Allgemeine Wiener medi-
cinische Zeitung* 3 (1858), 20:1 and 21:1. Skoda does assert that puerperal fever is
a kind of pyemia—he also said this in his 1849 lecture—but this is not conclusive
unless one can show that he also ascribed pyemia to a single necessary cause.

160. Lesky says this, op. cit., note 56 above, p. 186. In a recent paper, Sherwin
B. Nuland says the same thing: "Skoda and Rokitansky both recognized that the

Rokitansky probably regarded Semmelweis's logic as an incomprehensible and illegitimate mutation (as did everyone else), and while it may have borne a superficial resemblance to their own progeny, they neither could nor probably would have claimed any role in its paternity.

It is generally agreed that in later years neither Skoda nor Rokitansky ever mentioned Semmelweis in lectures or published works.[161] This curiosity is usually explained as a consequence of Semmelweis's abrupt departure from Vienna in 1850; Skoda and Rokitansky were, presumably, offended by his ingratitude and by his unwillingness to persist in seeking the recognition that they had consistently sought on his behalf.[162] But surely this explanation is inadequate. Even in lectures on puerperal fever Skoda not only failed to mention Semmelweis— he did not even adopt Semmelweis's most important theoretical innovation. It is hard to believe that a personal affront could have led Skoda to ignore something in these professional matters if he knew that it was true. The most plausible interpretation is that Skoda and Rokitansky, like everyone else, failed to see the value and justification for Semmelweis's innovation. They probably believed that associating themselves with a person who made such patently false and unjustifiable claims could only compro-

---

puerperal fever discovery was a logical outcome of their own teachings in the new methods of scientific logic. Erna Lesky . . . states that not only were these two rising giants the supporters of Semmelweis, but the 'intellectual fathers of his discovery.'" Op. cit., note 17 above, p. 257. Neither Nuland nor Lesky bothers to explain how Skoda and Rokitansky could recognize Semmelweis's theory as a logical outcome of their own teachings and at the same time fail to accept it.

161. See above, note 71.

162. This is the universal interpretation; Gortvay and Zoltán (ibid., pp. 72f.) and Lesky and Nuland (Nuland, op. cit., note 17 above, pp. 264f.) even agree on this. It is also part of the legend that "the Semmelweis theory of puerperal fever stood on the verge of acceptance" when Semmelweis suddenly abandoned the fight and returned to Budapest. Ibid., p. 264. The chlorine washings may have stood on the verge of acceptance, but there is no evidence whatsoever that anyone in Vienna ever understood the theory, much less was ready to accept it. Skoda, for example, still hadn't accepted the theory eight years later in 1858. See above, notes 158 and 159. The problem here, as with the endless debates regarding Semmelweis's priority, is that no one bothers to determine what the theory in question is, before deciding that Semmelweis didn't originate it or that the Viennese were on the verge of accepting it.

mise their own professional credibility. Thus they had to remain silent or reject that which they regarded as false. Had they entered into the discussion of 1850 or had they referred to his works in later years, they would have been obliged to reject those aspects of his work that they found objectionable. Since they seem never to have accepted his central idea that the disease could be recharacterized in terms of a necessary cause, if they had responded to his work they would probably have ended up saying the same things that Scanzoni, Braun, Lumpe, and all the others said. Perhaps they preferred simply to remain silent.

VII

It is difficult to determine precisely what impact Semmelweis had on his contemporaries. His use of chlorine was probably more influential, even during his lifetime, than he himself realized. Some of those who wrote to Semmelweis observed that his practices were influencing physicians throughout Europe, but that no one was willing to admit openly that this was the case.[163] If true, this was almost certainly because the practical results of Semmelweis's work continued to become progressively more obvious, while the theoretical basis for those results continued to appear speculative and false.

Because Joseph Lister's antiseptic procedures proved to be so famous and so successful, it would be of interest to determine whether he was influenced by Semmelweis. As early as 1894 Lister was quoted as having said, "Without Semmelweis I could not have succeeded, modern surgery owes much to that great Hungarian."[164] But Lister himself denied having made this statement, and intensive investigation suggests that the statement is probably spurious.[165] Lister's own account of his relation to Semmelweis is contained in a letter that was written on 2 April 1906: "When in 1865 I applied the principles of antisepsis to the treatment of wounds the name of Semmelweis was not yet familiar to me, and I confess, I had not even heard of his work.

163. See below, p. 186; German edition, pp. 306f.
164. Gortvay and Zoltán, op. cit., note 1 above, p. 220.
165. Ibid., pp. 220–22.

When twenty years later I visited Budapest, I was received with the warmest welcome both by colleagues and university students, and even at that occasion the name of Semmelweis was not mentioned, he seems to have been forgotten by his native country to the same extent as by everybody else throughout the world. It was much later that a Hungarian physician in London of the name of Dr. [Theodor] Duka, had called my attention to Semmelweis and his work. Although Semmelweis never influenced my own work, I think with the greatest admiration of him and his achievement and it fills me with joy that at last he is given the respect due to him."[166] There is a good possibility that Lister did hear of Semmelweis, however; at least he had several opportunities to do so. First, while Lister was a student, Semmelweis was often mentioned in British medical literature.[167] Furthermore, M. J. Duncan, who was Simpson's assistant and who may have persuaded Simpson to adopt Semmelweis's methods, had intimate ties with Lister.[168] When Lister married in 1856, he and his wife spent two weeks in Vienna. At that time they were guests in Rokitansky's home, and Rokitansky spent over three hours showing Lister his medical museum.[169] This was just about the time that Rokitansky and others in Vienna were recommending Semmelweis as the successor to Johann Klein, who had died in the same year.[170] Second, Lister spent three days in Budapest in 1883; by this time he had become famous for his work on antisepsis. Lister spent one long evening at a large public gathering at which Dr. Lajos Markusovszky presided.[171] Markusovszky, a lifelong friend and colleague of Semmelweis's, may have been among the few persons in Europe

166. Ibid., pp. 220f.

167. See above, note 107.

168. Gortvay and Zoltán, op. cit., note 1 above, p. 223.

169. Owen H. Wangensteen, "Nineteenth-Century Wound Management of the Parturient Uterus and Compound Fracture: The Semmelweis-Lister Priority Controversy." *Bulletin of the New York Academy of Medicine* 46 (1970), 464–596: 586.

170. Lesky, op. cit., note 63 above, pp. 83–93.

171. Owen H. Wangensteen and Sarah D. Wangensteen, "Lister's Books and the Evolvement of Antiseptic Wound Practices," *Bulletin of the History of Medicine* 48 (1974), 106–132: 120f.

who understood and agreed with Semmelweis's theoretical approach in dealing with puerperal fever. Owen H. and Sarah D. Wangensteen called attention to a copy of Semmelweis's *Aetiologie* bearing the signature of Lajos Markusovszky that is now in the library of the Wellcome Institute in London. They suggest that this book may have been sent to Lister sometime after his visit to Budapest.[172] It would have been very natural for Semmelweis to have been mentioned in either of these contexts.

In 1896 Lister finally abandoned his earlier procedures that involved wound irrigation and adopted instead prophylactic antiseptic practices—basically the same practices that Semmelweis had advocated. The Wangensteens conclude that Lister certainly knew and was influenced by the work of Semmelweis in making this change.[173]

It would also be significant if one could show that Semmelweis's theoretical approach influenced subsequent work in medical theory. It is generally agreed that the move toward etiological characterizations of specific diseases was one facet of a nineteenth-century revolution in medical thought. This revolution has generally been associated with bacteriology. After noting that the work of Koch and Pasteur enabled physicians to adopt new characterizations of diseases in terms of specific microorganisms rather than in terms of morbid anatomical modifications, Owsei Temkin writes, "Although bacteriology concerned infectious diseases only, its influence on the general concept of disease was great. Presumably, diseases could be bound to definite causes; hence the knowledge of the cause was needed to elevate a clinical entity or a syndrome to the rank of a disease."[174] As we have seen, this approach existed in medicine quite apart from any serious interest in microorganisms. In fact, however, neither Koch nor Pasteur ever mentioned Semmelweis in their published works. There seem to be only tenuous and indirect connections between Semmelweis and either of them.[175]

172. Ibid., pp. 119f.

173. Ibid., p. 124.

174. Owsei Temkin, "Health and Disease," reprinted in *The Double Face of Janus* (Baltimore: Johns Hopkins University Press, 1977), p. 436.

175. For example, in his discussion of the etiology of infected wound diseases,

VIII

After returning to Budapest in 1850 Semmelweis was appointed as an unpaid director of the obstetrical clinic at the St. Rochus hospital. At that time the clinic was seriously troubled with childbed fever. Semmelweis achieved results similar to those achieved in the first clinic in Vienna. Even in Budapest, however, many of his colleagues seem not to have been persuaded by his success. Ede Flórián Birly, who was Professor of Obstetrics at the University of Pest while Semmelweis was working at the St. Rochus hospital, never adopted Semmelweis's methods, and when Birly died and the medical faculty was seeking his successor, Semmelweis received fewer votes than did Carl Braun, Semmelweis's arch rival and antagonist.[176]

In 1857 Semmelweis married Mária Weidinhoffer (1837–1910), a daughter of a successful merchant in Pest. In the same year they were married, he received a call to become professor of obstetrics at the University of Zurich,[177] but decided to remain in Budapest. During these years Semmelweis was active in various projects. In addition to his publications on puerperal fever, he helped to found and also contributed several articles to a Hungarian medical periodical. He began writing a handbook of obstetrics. He was also active on various university committees, and functioned as the economic superintendent of the medical

---

Robert Koch gives considerable attention to puerperal fever. He bases this part of the discussion on Wilhelm Waldeyer. Robert Koch, "Untersuchungen über die Aetiologie der Wundinfektionskrankheiten," reprinted in Julius Schwalbe (ed.), *Gesammelte Werke von Robert Koch* (Leipzig: Georg Thieme, 1912), vol. 1, pp. 61–108. Waldeyer, in turn, cites Karl Meyrhofer. "Über das Vorkommen von Bacterien bei der diphtheritischen Form des Puerperalfiebers," *Archiv für Gynaekologie* 3 (1872), 293–306: 294. Meyrhofer wrote a series of papers between 1863 and 1865 in which he argued that a specific form of microorganism constituted a necessary cause for puerperal fever. The most complete paper was "Zur Frage nach der Aetiologie der Puerperalprocesse," *Monatsschrift für Geburtskunde und Frauenkrankheiten* 25 (1865), 112–34. At the time he wrote these papers, Meyrhofer was an assistant in the Viennese Obstetrical Clinic, and he must have known of Semmelweis. Meyrhofer, however, never mentioned Semmelweis in his papers. This may have been because at this time Carl Braun was Meyrhofer's chief.

176. Gortvay and Zoltán, op. cit., note 1 above, pp. 91–93.
177. Ibid., pp. 100f.

faculty. When his writings did not convince the medical world, he also wrote a series of open letters to various prominent obstetricians.[178] The open letters were highly polemical and superlatively offensive; they probably did little to persuade those to whom they were addressed. By the time of their publication, however, Semmelweis's prophylactic measures were probably beginning to influence medical thought rather significantly.[179]

Beginning about 1861 Semmelweis suffered from nervous complaints. As time progressed he became irritable and was easily excitable; he suffered from severe depression and he became excessively absentminded. Paintings of Semmelweis over the years from 1857 to 1864 show that he aged very rapidly.[180] In July 1865 it was his duty to read a report in a faculty meeting. Semmelweis's former assistant József Fleischer relates that when he was called on to do so "he rose, took a piece of paper from his trouser pocket and, to the stupefication of those present, began to read the text of the midwives' oath."[181] There was no doubt about his condition, and his colleagues took him home. "This was the last function he performed in his faculty, which had lost the most accomplished, and the most illustrious of its professors."[182]

Semmelweis was taken by train to Vienna where he was met by Professor Hebra. He was taken to the Lower-Austrian Mental Home and was confined to the ward for maniacs. The following day his wife visited the home to see him, but she was told that the night before Semmelweis had tried to get out and that it had required six attendants to hold him back. She was not allowed to see him. Within two weeks, on 13 August 1865, Semmelweis died.

Much has been written about the nature of Semmelweis's ill-

---

178. The letters are reprinted in Győry, op. cit., note 59 above, pp. 429–511.

179. Gortvay and Zoltán, op. cit., note 1 above, pp. 170–72. By 1864 Josef Späth, who had been among the outspoken critics of Semmelweis's ideas endorsed at least the practical measures suggested by those ideas. Murphy, op. cit., note 2 above, pp. 669f.

180. Gortvay and Zoltán, op. cit., note 1 above, pp. 6, 183–86.

181. Ibid., p. 187.

182. Ibid.

ness and about the cause of his death. In particular, it is usually reported that he died from pyemia, possibly because of a wound incurred during an autopsy just before his breakdown. After a review of the evidence, Sherwin B. Nuland recently concluded that Semmelweis probably suffered from Alzheimer's disease— a form of presenile dementia, the most prominent characteristics of which are deterioration of intellect, failure of memory, and a striking appearance of rapid aging.[183] Nuland also concludes that Semmelweis died of wounds inflicted when he was forcibly restrained by the attendants at the mental home—that he was, in effect, beaten to death.

Semmelweis's remains were originally buried in Vienna, but in 1891 they were transferred to Budapest. On 11 October 1964 they were transferred once more to a space in the garden wall of the house in which he was born. The house, in the meantime, had been converted into an historical museum and library, a monument to Ignaz Semmelweis, one of Hungary's most brilliant sons.

183. Nuland, op. cit., note 17, p. 270.

*The Etiology, Concept, and
Prophylaxis of Childbed Fever*

by

Ignaz Philipp Semmelweis

Doctor of Medicine and Surgery, Master of Obstetrics,
Professor of Theoretical and Practical Obstetrics
at the Royal Hungarian University of Pest

Preface

After twice completing the course in practical obstetrics at the first maternity clinic in Vienna, I presented myself on 1 July 1844 to the director of the clinic, the late Professor Dr. [Johann] Klein,[1] as a candidate for a future post of assistant physician at the clinic. I was provisionally appointed to this post by a decree dated 27 February 1846. On 1 July 1846 I officially assumed the position of assistant at the first maternity clinic. On 20 October of the same year, however, I was obliged to withdraw in favor of my predecessor, Dr. [Franz] Breit, because Dr. Breit had in the meantime received a two-year extension of his service. That I may be understood, in the course of this essay I will refer to these four months, namely July, August, September, and October of 1846, as my first period of service. *[iv]* In Vienna, the period of service of the assistants in all departments was fixed at two years. In every other department it was customary, after the expiration of two years, for the appointment to be extended for an additional two years. In the obstetrical department this had not been the practice, however, and the assistants were regularly changed every two years. Dr. Breit was the first to enjoy this privilege [of a two-year extension]. Then Dr. Breit was named Professor of Obstetrics at the medical school at Tübingen, and for the second time I officially assumed the position of assistant, on 20 March 1847. I functioned as such for two years, until 20 March 1849. I refer to these two years as my second period of service.

The object of this essay is this: to present historically to the medical instructor observations that I made at this clinic in this period, to demonstrate how I began to doubt existing teachings concerning the origin and the concept of childbed fever, and how

1. Johann Klein (1788–1856) was Professor of Obstetrics at the University of Salzburg and at the University of Vienna. As Semmelweis's chief in the maternity clinic, he seems to have felt threatened by the younger members of the faculty, and he opposed both Semmelweis and his theories.

I was irresistibly forced to my present conviction, in order that he also, for the welfare of mankind, may derive the same convictions.

[v] By nature I am averse to all polemics. This is proven by my having left numerous attacks unanswered. I believed that I could leave it to time to break a path for the truth. However, for thirteen years my expectations have not been fulfilled to the degree that is essential for the well-being of mankind. An additional misfortune was that in the school years of 1856–57 and 1857–58, maternity patients died in such numbers at my own obstetrical clinic in Pest that my opponents could use these deaths as evidence against me. It must be shown that these two unfortunate years provide tragic and unintentional yet direct confirmation of my views.

To my aversion to all polemics must be added my innate aversion to every form of writing. Fate has chosen me as the representative of those truths that are laid down in this essay. It is my inescapable obligation to support them. I have given up the hope that the importance and the truth of the matter would make all controversy unnecessary. Rather than my inclinations, people's lives must be considered, people who do not even participate in the conflict over whether my opponents or I have the truth. *[vi]* Since silence has proven futile, I must forcibly restrain my inclinations and step once more before the public as though uncautioned by the many bitter hours I have endured. I have made the best of these hours; for those yet to come I find consolation in knowing that I advocate only that which is firmly grounded in my own convictions.

Pest, 30 August 1860

CHAPTER I

Autobiographical Introduction

[1] Medicine's highest duty is saving threatened human life, and obstetrics is the branch of medicine in which this duty is most obviously fulfilled. Frequently it is necessary to deliver a child in transverse lie. Mother and child will probably die if the birth is left to nature, while the obstetrician's timely helping hand, almost painlessly and taking only a few minutes, can save both.

I was already familiar with this prerogative of obstetrics from the theoretical lectures on the specialty. I found it perfectly confirmed as I had the opportunity to learn the practical aspects of obstetrics in the large Viennese maternity hospital. But unfortunately the number of cases in which the obstetrician achieves such blessings vanishes in comparison with the number of victims to whom his help is of no avail. This dark side of obstetrics is childbed fever. Each year I saw ten or fifteen crises in which the salvation of mother and child could be achieved. I also saw many hundreds of maternity patients treated unsuccessfully for childbed fever. *[2]* Not only was therapy unsuccessful, the etiology seemed deficient. The accepted etiology of childbed fever, on the basis of which I saw so many hundreds of maternity patients treated unsuccessfully, cannot contain the actual causal factor of the disease.

The large gratis Viennese maternity hospital is divided into two clinics; one is called the first, the other the second. By Imperial Decree of 10 October 1840, Court Commission for Education Decree of 17 October 1840, and Administrative Ordinance of 27 October 1840, all male students were assigned to the first clinic and all female students to the second. Before this time student obstetricians and midwives received training in equal numbers in both clinics.

[3] TABLE 1

	First Clinic			Second Clinic		
	Births	Deaths	Rate	Births	Deaths	Rate
1841	3,036	237	7.7	2,442	86	3.5
1842	3,287	518	15.8	2,659	202	7.5
1843	3,060	274	8.9	2,739	164	5.9
1844	3,157	260	8.2	2,956	68	2.3
1845	3,492	241	6.8	3,241	66	2.03
1846	4,010	459	11.4	3,754	105	2.7
Total	20,042	1,989		17,791	691	
Avg.			9.92			3.38

The admission of maternity patients was regulated as follows: Monday afternoon at four o'clock admissions began in the first clinic and continued until Tuesday afternoon at four. Admissions then began in the second clinic and continued until Wednesday afternoon at four o'clock. At that time admissions were resumed in the first clinic until Thursday afternoon, etc. On Friday afternoon at four o'clock admissions began in the first clinic and continued through forty-eight hours until Sunday afternoon, at which time admissions began again in the second clinic. Admissions alternated between the two clinics through twenty-four hour periods, and only once a week did admissions continue in the first clinic for forty-eight hours. Thus the first clinic admitted patients four days a week, whereas the second clinic admitted for only three days. The first clinic, thereby, had fifty-two more days of admissions [each year] than the second.

[3] From the time the first clinic began training only obstetricians until June 1847, the mortality rate in the first clinic was consistently greater than in the second clinic, where only midwives were trained. Indeed, in the year 1846, the mortality rate in the first clinic was five times as great as in the second, and through a six-year period it was, on the average, three times as great. This is shown in Table 1.

The difference in mortality between the clinics was actually larger than the table suggests, because occasionally, for reasons to be examined later,[1] during times of high mortality all ill maternity patients in the first clinic were transferred to the general hospital. When these patients died, they were included in the mortality figures for the general hospital rather than for the maternity hospital. When the transfers were undertaken, the reports show reduced mortality, since only those who could not be transferred because of the rapid course of their illness were included. In reality, many additional victims should be included. [4] In the second clinic such transfers were never undertaken. Only isolated patients were transferred whose condition might endanger the other patients.

The additional mortality in the first clinic consisted of many hundreds of maternity patients, some of whom I saw die from puerperal processes, but for whose deaths I could find no explanation in the existing etiology. To convince the reader that this additional mortality cannot be explained by the existing etiology, we must examine more carefully the previously acknowledged causes of childbed fever that have been used in attempting to explain this additional mortality.

It has not been questioned and has been expressed thousands of times that the horrible ravages of childbed fever are caused by epidemic influences. By epidemic influences one understands atmospheric-cosmic-terrestrial changes,[2] as yet not precisely defined, that often extend over whole countrysides, and by which childbed fever is generated in persons predisposed by the puerperal state. But if the atmospheric-cosmic-terrestrial conditions of Vienna cause puerperal fever in predisposed persons, how is it that for many years these conditions have affected persons in the first clinic while sparing similarly predisposed persons in the second? [5] To me there appears no doubt that if the ravages of childbed fever in the first clinic are caused by epidemic influ-

1. See below, pp. 73, 83f.; German edition, pp. 35, 48.
2. Physicians actually used the phrase "atmospheric-cosmic-terrestrial [or telluric] influences." See, for example, p. 343 of Eduard Caspar Jakob von Siebold, "Betrachtungen über das Kindbettfieber," *Monatsschrift für Geburtskunde und Frauenkrankheiten* 17(1861), 335–57, 401–17, and 18, 19–39; and pp. 255–58 of Anselm Martin, "Zur Erforschung der Ursachen des epidemischen Puerperalfiebers," ibid. 10(1857), 253–73.

ences, the same conditions must operate with minimal variation in the second clinic. Otherwise, one is forced to the unreasonable assumption that lethal epidemic influences undergo twenty-four-hour remissions and exacerbations and that the remissions, through a series of years, have exactly coincided with admissions to the second clinic, while the exacerbations begin precisely at the time of admission to the first clinic.

However, even with such unreasonable assumptions, epidemic influences cannot explain the differences in mortality. The exacerbated influences must affect individuals either before they are admitted to the maternity hospital or during their stay. If they operate outside the hospital, certainly those who are admitted to the first clinic will be no more subject to them than those admitted to the second. No significant difference in mortality between the equally exposed patients admitted to the two clinics would then exist. On the other hand, if epidemic influences operate on individuals during their stay in the hospital, there could be no difference in the mortality rate, since two clinics so near one another that they share a common anteroom must necessarily be subject to the same atmospheric-cosmic-terrestrial influences. [6] These considerations alone forced me to the unshakable conviction that epidemic influences were not responsible for the horrible devastations of the maternity patients in the first clinic.

Once I had come to this conviction, other supporting considerations occurred to me. If the atmospheric influences of Vienna occasion an epidemic in the maternity hospital, then necessarily there must be an epidemic among maternity patients throughout Vienna because the entire population is subject to the same influences. But in fact, while the puerperal disease rages most furiously in the maternity hospital, it is only infrequently observed either in Vienna at large or in the surrounding countryside. During a cholera epidemic, people in general are affected, not just those in a particular hospital. A common and successful expedient for halting an epidemic of childbed fever is to close the maternity hospitals. Hospitals are closed not to force maternity patients to die somewhere else, but because of the belief that if patients deliver in the hospital they are subject to epidemic influences, whereas if they deliver elsewhere they will remain healthy. However, this proves one is not dealing with a disease dependent on atmospheric influences, because these influences would extend beyond the hospital into every part of the city. *[7]* This proves that the disease is endemic—a disease due to causes limited by the boundaries of the hospital. What would defenders of the epidemic conception say if someone proposed to control cholera by closing cholera hospitals? Puerperal fever that originates traumatically, for example, in a forced delivery by forceps, is entirely the same in its course and in its anatomical manifestations as the so-called epidemic form. Can any other epidemic disease be generated by trauma? Epidemics exhibit intermissions perhaps years in duration; childbed fever has ravaged the first clinic for years without even minimal intermissions. Do cholera epidemics occur annually? If so-called childbed fever epidemics were really due to atmospheric influences, then they could not occur in opposing seasons and climates. In actual fact, however, the disease is observed in all seasons, in the most different climates, and under all weather conditions.

To prove numerically that seasons have no influence on the incidence of childbed fever, I will utilize the time interval represented in Table 1, together with the first five months of 1847. This will prove that every month of the year can be either favorable or unfavorable for the health of patients in the first clinic. I omit only December 1841, since I have lost the figures for this month. *[8]* However, this month may belong to those in which many patients died, since it is between other months in which patients were unhealthy. In November 1841, 53 of 235 patients died (22.55 percent), and in January 1842, 64 of 307 died (20.84 percent). This is shown in Table 2.

[9–10] The reader will observe that epidemic influences are so powerful that their pernicious activity cannot be restricted to a particular season. They rage with equal violence in the bitterest cold of winter and in the oppressive heat of summer, but they do not scourge all maternity hospitals equally; they spare some while raging all the more furiously in others. Indeed, they are so partial that they afflict differently the different divisions of the same institution.

[9] TABLE 2

	Lowest Mortality				Highest Mortality			
	Year	Births	Deaths	Rate	Year	Births	Deaths	Rate
Jan.	1847	311	10	3.21	1842	307	64	20.84
Feb.	1847	312	6	1.92	1846	293	53	18.08
Mar.	1847	305	11	3.60	1846	311	48	15.43
Apr.	1841	255	4	1.57	1846	253	48	18.97
May	1841	255	2	0.74	1846	305	41	13.44
Jun.	1844	224	6	2.67	1846	266	27	10.15
Jul.	1843	191	1	0.52	1842	231	48	20.79
Aug.	1841	222	3	1.35	1842	216	55	25.46
Sept.	1844	245	3	1.22	1842	223	41	18.38
Oct.	1844	248	8	3.22	1842	242	71	29.33
Nov.	1843	252	18	7.14	1841	235	53	22.55
Dec.	1846	298	16	5.37	1842	239	75	31.38

With a few exceptions, maternity hospitals that are not teaching institutions or that train only midwives are more favorable than institutions that train obstetricians. Table 1 shows the different mortality rates of two divisions of one institution; a similar difference occurred in the two divisions of the maternity hospital at Strasbourg. Later we will speak more of these circumstances.[3]

As explained before, these considerations strengthened my conviction that the great mortality of the first clinic was not due to epidemic influences but rather to harmful endemic factors (i.e., to a cause manifested so horribly only within the first clinic). However, when we examine the previously acknowledged endemic causes in reference to the comparative mortality rates of the two clinics, we see either that no difference in mortality could exist or that the second clinic must have the larger rate. *[11]* If overcrowding were the cause of death, mortality in the second clinic would have been larger, because the second clinic was more crowded than the first. Because of the bad reputation of the first clinic, everyone sought admission to the second clinic. For this reason, the second clinic was often unable to resume admissions at the specified time because it was impossible to accommodate new arrivals. Or if the second clinic began to admit, within a few hours it was necessary to resume admitting patients to the first clinic because the passageway was crowded with such a great number of persons awaiting admission to the second clinic. In a short time all the free places were taken. In the five years I was associated with the first clinic, not once did overcrowding make it necessary to reopen admission to the second clinic. This was true even though once each week the first clinic admitted continuously for a period of forty-eight hours. In spite of this overcrowding, the mortality rate in the second clinic was strikingly smaller.

Each year, the first clinic recorded hundreds more births than the second. This, however, was because each week it had one more day of admissions and had, therefore, a larger assigned area. In spite of its smaller number of births with respect to its

3. See below, pp. 126–28; German edition, pp. 131–35.

capacity, the second clinic was more crowded. *[12]* This is ver-
ified by the fact that the second clinic was often unable to resume
admissions or had to discontinue admissions early, which never
happened at the first clinic. Had the second clinic been large
enough to admit all who sought admission, it would have had
significantly more births each year than the first clinic, even
though it had fifty-two fewer days of admissions. If we disregard the comparative overcrowding within the two clinics, and
consider only the degree of overcrowding within the first clinic
as determined by the number of patients treated within a given
month, it is apparent than the favorable or unfavorable health of
the patients was not due to the degree of overcrowding. Again I
use the time interval of Table 1, together with the first five months
of 1847. Mortality in these months is shown in Table 3. [Sem-
melweis gives eighteen pages of further tables presenting this
information in different arrangements. He then continues:]

[13–32] One may believe that a location in which so many
thousands of individuals have given birth, contracted childbed
fever, and died must inevitably be so infested that the presence
of childbed fever is no surprise. If this were the case, however,
the mortality in the second clinic would be greater, since in the
location of the second clinic, even in [Rogers Lucas Johann] Boër's
times,[4] serious epidemics of puerperal fever raged. At that time,
the building now occupied by the first clinic was not even built.

It has been proposed that the evil reputation of the institution,
with its great annual contingent of deaths, so frightens the newly
admitted patients that they become ill and die. The patients really
do fear the first clinic. Frequently one must witness moving scenes
in which patients, kneeling and wringing their hands, beg to be
released in order to seek admission to the second clinic. Such
persons have usually been admitted because they are ignorant of
the reputation of the first clinic, but they soon become suspi-
cious because of the large number of doctors present. *[33]* One

4. Rogers Lucas Johann Boër (1751–1835) was the first professor of obstetrics
at the Viennese maternity hospital; he served from 1789 until 1822. He was an
outstanding advocate of the conservative trend in obstetrics. He strongly discouraged use of forceps and other instruments and advocated the practice of
natural parturition.

sees maternity patients with abnormally high pulse rates, bloated stomachs, and dry tongues (in other words, very ill with puerperal fever), still insisting only hours before death that they are perfectly healthy, because they know that treatment by the physicians is the forerunner of death. Nevertheless, I could not convince myself that fear was the cause of the high mortality rate in the first clinic. As a physician, I could not understand how fear, a psychological condition, could bring about such physical changes as occur in childbed fever. Moreover, it would have required a long period of time with consistently unequal mortality rates for ordinary people, who did not have access to hospital reports, to become aware that one clinic had a much greater mortality rate than the other. Fear could not account for the initial difference.

Even religious practices did not escape attention. The hospital chapel was so located that when the priest was summoned to administer last rites in the second clinic, he could go directly to the room set aside for ill patients. On the other hand, when he was summoned to the first clinic he had to pass through five other rooms because the room containing ill patients was sixth in line from the chapel. According to accepted Catholic practice, when visiting the sick to administer last rites, the priest generally arrived in ornate vestments and was preceded by a sacristan who rang a bell. This was supposed to occur only once in twenty-four hours. Yet twenty-four hours is a long time for someone suffering from childbed fever. Many who appeared tolerably healthy at the time of the priest's visit, and who therefore did not require last rites, were so ill a few hours later that the priest had to be summoned again. *[34]* One can imagine the impression that was created on the other patients when the priest came several times a day, each time accompanied by the clearly audible bell. Even to me it was very demoralizing to hear the bell hurry past my door. I groaned within for the victim who had fallen to an unknown cause. The bell was a painful admonition to seek this unknown cause with all my powers. It had been proposed that even this difference in the two clinics explained the different mortality rates. During my first period of service, I appealed to the compassion of the servant of God and arranged for him to come by a less direct route, without bells, and without passing

[13] TABLE 3

	1841			1842			1843		
	Births	Deaths	Rate	Births	Deaths	Rate	Births	Deaths	R:
Jan.	254	37	14.56	307	64	20.84	272	52	19
Feb.	239	18	7.53	311	38	12.21	263	42	15
Mar.	277	12	4.33	264	27	10.23	266	33	12
Apr.	255	4	1.57	242	26	10.74	285	34	11
May	255	2	0.78	310	10	3.22	246	15	6
Jun.	200	10	5.00	273	18	6.60	196	8	4
Jul.	190	16	8.42	231	48	20.79	191	1	0
Aug.	222	3	1.35	216	55	25.46	193	3	1
Sept.	213	4	1.87	223	41	18.38	221	5	2
Oct.	236	26	11.00	242	71	29.33	250	44	17
Nov.	235	53	22.55	209	48	22.96	252	18	7
Dec.				239	75	31.38	236	19	8

	1844			1845			1846		
	Births	Deaths	Rate	Births	Deaths	Rate	Births	Deaths	R
Jan.	244	37	15.16	303	23	7.59	336	45	1:
Feb.	257	29	11.28	274	13	5.11	293	53	18
Mar.	276	47	17.03	292	13	4.45	311	48	15
Apr.	208	36	17.80	260	11	4.23	253	48	18
May	240	14	5.83	296	13	4.39	305	41	1:
Jun.	224	6	2.67	280	20	7.14	266	27	1(
Jul.	206	9	4.37	245	15	6.12	252	33	1:
Aug.	269	17	6.32	251	9	3.58	216	39	18
Sept.	245	3	1.22	237	25	10.55	271	39	1<
Oct.	248	8	3.22	283	42	14.84	254	38	1<
Nov.	245	27	11.00	265	29	10.94	297	32	1(
Dec.	256	27	10.55	267	28	10.48	298	16	:

1847		
Births	Deaths	Rate
311	10	3.21
312	6	1.92
305	11	3.60
312	57	18.27
294	36	12.24
268	6	2.38
250	3	1.20
264	5	1.89
262	12	5.23
278	11	3.95
246	11	4.47
273	8	2.93

through the other clinic rooms. Thus, no one outside the room containing the ill patients knew of the priest's presence. The two clinics were made identical in this respect as well, but the mortality rate was unaffected.

The high mortality was also attributed to the clinic's practice of admitting only single women in desperate circumstances. These women had been obliged throughout their pregnancies to support themselves by working hard. They were miserable and in great need, often malnourished, and may have attempted to induce miscarriages. But if these conditions constituted the cause, the mortality rate in the second clinic should have been the same, since the same type of women were admitted there.

It had also been proposed that the high mortality rate in the first clinic resulted from the obstetricians examining the patients in a rougher manner than did the student midwives. *[35]* If inserting the finger, however roughly, into the vagina and to the adjacent parts of the uterus—already widened and extended by pregnancy—was sufficient to cause damages leading to so horrible a condition, then surely the passage of the baby's body through the birth canal must cause damage so much worse that every birth would end in the death of the mother.

It had also been suggested that the mortality rate in the first clinic resulted from the offense to modesty incurred through the presence of males at delivery. As those familiar with the Viennese maternity hospital realize, patients are troubled by fear but not by offended modesty. Moreover, it is not clear how this offended modesty would bring about the exudative mortal processes of the disease.

Since they were the same in both clinics, medical procedures were not responsible for the increased death rate. Also, as part of an experiment, all diseased maternity patients were occasionally transferred to the general hospital. They succumbed there after very different treatments. It was not that equal numbers became ill and fewer recovered in the first clinic than in the second. Rather, more patients became ill in the first clinic. The recovery rate in both clinics was the same. *[36]* However, obstetrical practices, numerous and rough procedures, etc., did not cause a great number of illnesses in the first clinic, because the majority of those who became ill had not been subjected to special obstetrical procedures. In both divisions, patients were treated according to Boër's principles.[5]

In the first clinic it was the custom that three hours after giving birth, patients would get up from the delivery bed and walk through a passageway to their own beds. The passageway was enclosed in glass and was heated in the winter. This was a considerable distance for those whose beds were furthest from the delivery room. Nevertheless, only those who were weak or ill or had had special operations were carried.[6] But this inconvenience was not responsible for the greater mortality rate, since the second clinic was subject to the same drawback. Indeed, circumstances were worse there, since the second clinic was divided by a common unheated anteroom and patients whose beds were in rooms beyond the anteroom had to walk through that as well.

In the first clinic, a large maternity room on the third floor was reached through a glass-enclosed stairway. Since one could not expect newly delivered patients to go there on foot, it was necessary for healthy patients to be transferred there seven or eight days after delivery. At that time they would normally have been allowed to leave their beds in any case. This second move did not cause the greater mortality rate, since after seven or eight

5. "In 1723 forceps had come into general use. Delighted with the beneficial invention, French and German obstetricians (Osiander) applied them on every occasion, even when there was no need for them. One might have thought that 'Nature had abandoned its delivery job and left it to the obstetrician's instrument' (Boër). Against this busy use of instruments Boër employed his patient procedure of waiting and relying on the natural forces of the organism. In limiting instrumental and manual intervention to the cases in which such assistance was indicated and in 'restoring the delivery power of Nature to its rights,' he became the founder of the new obstetrical natural method." Erna Lesky, *The Vienna Medical School of the Nineteenth Century* (Baltimore: Johns Hopkins University Press, 1976), p. 52.

6. Lajos Markusovszky, Semmelweis's close friend and associate, recorded that Semmelweis had newly delivered patients carried back to their beds so that they would not be obliged to walk. György Gortvay and Imre Zoltán, *Semmelweis: His Life and Work* (Budapest: Akadémiai Kiadó, 1968), p. 48.

days patients seldom became ill. Moreover, the second clinic followed exactly the same procedure.

[37] Poor ventilation in the first clinic, which even in winter was for the most part accomplished by opening windows, was also proposed as an explanation for the more numerous deaths in the first clinic. Those making this proposal overlooked the fact that the second clinic was ventilated in the same way. The laundry process was blamed because the contractor mixed the laundry with that of the general hospital. Yet laundry from the second clinic was mixed in just the same way. The disadvantage of being in close contact with so large a hospital as the Viennese Imperial General Hospital was also shared by both clinics. Indeed, the clinics were so close that they shared a common anteroom and were constructed in a similar fashion. Other disadvantages, such as continuous use for instructional purposes, free passage between wards for sick and well patients, unrestricted contact between attendants for the sick and those for the healthy, were also shared by both clinics. Neither catching a cold nor errors in diet could explain the differences in mortality between the two clinics. The possibility of contracting colds was the same in both, and the food in both clinics conformed to the same dietary standards and was prepared by the same contractor.

These are the endemic causes to which was attributed the greater mortality among maternity patients in the first clinic. [38] With the exception of one circumstance which will be discussed later, I fully agree that these do not adequately explain the greater mortality in the first clinic. We have shown that these harmful endemic factors were either equally operative in both clinics, in which case mortality would have been the same, or they were more pronounced in the second clinic than in the first, in which case the second clinic should have had more deaths. However, precisely the opposite has regularly occurred. Since the first clinic has been used exclusively for training obstetricians, its mortality rate has consistently been significantly greater than that of the second clinic.

Since neither epidemic influences nor the previously acknowledged endemic factors can explain the greater mortality rate of the first clinic, we must consider other factors that have been proposed as causes of childbed fever.

Recent investigators blame the disease on the most remote of all possible causes—conception itself. Supposedly, the penetration of sperm occasions a manifold series of alterations, including partially unknown changes in the blood. But I suspect that I am not misinformed in claiming that those who delivered in the second clinic must also have conceived. What is the origin, then, of the difference in mortality between the clinics? *[39]* Hyperinosis [excessive fibrin in the blood], hydremia [excessive water in the blood], plethora [an excessive quantity of blood], disturbances caused by the pregnant uterus, stagnation of the circulation, inopexia [spontaneous coagulation of the blood], delivery itself, decreased weight caused by the emptying of the uterus, protracted labor, wounding of the inner surface of the uterus in delivery, imperfect contractions, faulty involutions of the uterus during maternity, scanty and discontinued secretion and excretion of lochia [a vaginal discharge during the first few weeks after delivery], the weight of secreted milk, death of the fetus, and the individuality of patients are causes to which may be ascribed much or little influence in the generation of childbed fever. But in both clinics these must be equally harmful or harmless and they cannot, therefore, explain the appalling difference in mortality between the clinics.

While I was still unable to find a cause for the increased mortality rate in the first clinic, I became aware of other inexplicable circumstances. Those whose period of dilation was extended over twenty-four hours or more almost invariably became ill either immediately during birth or within the first twenty-four or thirty-six hours after delivery. They died quickly of rapidly developing childbed fever. An equally extended period of dilation in the second clinic did not prove dangerous. Because dilation was usually extended during first deliveries, those delivering for the first time usually died. I often pointed out to my students that because these blossoming, vigorously healthy young women had extended periods of dilation, they would die quickly from puerperal fever either during delivery or immediately thereafter. *[40]* My prognoses were fulfilled. I did not know why, but I often saw it happen. This circumstance was inexplicable, since it was not repeated in the second clinic. I speak here of the period of dilation, not of delivery; thus the trauma of delivery is not under consideration.

Not only these mothers but also their newborn infants, both male and female, died of childbed fever. I am not alone in speaking of puerperal fever of the newborn.[7] With the exception of the genital areas, the anatomical lesions in the corpses of such newborn infants are the same as the lesions in the corpses of women who die of puerperal fever. To recognize these findings as the consequence of puerperal fever in maternity patients but to deny that identical findings in the corpses of the newborn are the consequence of the same disease is to reject pathological anatomy.

But if the maternity patients and the newborn die from the same disease, then the etiology that accounts for the deaths of the mothers must also account for the deaths of the newborn. Since the difference in mortality between the maternity patients in the two clinics was reflected in the mortality rates for the newborn, the accepted etiology for childbed fever no more accounts for the deaths of the newborn than for the deaths of the maternity patients. Table 4 gives the mortality rates of the newborn at the two clinics.

[41] Because their mothers died or were otherwise unable to nurse, many of the newborn were sent directly to the foundling home. Later we will consider their fate.[8]

The occurrence of childbed fever among the newborn can be explained in two ways. Childbed fever may be caused by factors operating on the mother during the intrauterine life of the fetus,

7. Semmelweis was not alone, but he was in the minority. There was a discussion of infant puerperal fever in French medical literature in 1855. The discussion was reviewed in the *Monatsschrift für Geburtshülfe* 7(1856): 152f., and in the *Wiener medizinische Wochenschrift, Journal Revue*, no. 3 (1856): 22f. Carl Braun also mentioned that "the unmistakable influence of puerperal fever epidemics on the mortality of fetuses has been recognized in the Viennese maternity hospital for years"; he then notes that the French refer to such cases as puerperal fever of fetuses. Carl Braun, *Lehrbuch der Geburtshülfe* (Vienna: Braumüller, 1857), pp. 589f.

8. See below, pp. 99f.; German edition, pp. 67–69.

	First Clinic			Second Clinic		
	Births	Deaths	Rate	Births	Deaths	Rate
1841	2,813	177	6.2	2,252	91	4.04
1842	3,037	279	9.1	2,414	113	4.06
1843	2,828	195	6.8	2,570	130	5.05
1844	2,917	251	8.6	2,739	100	3.06
1845	3,201	260	8.1	3,017	97	3.02
1846	3,533	235	6.5	3,398	86	2.05

and the mother can then impart the disease to the infant. Alternatively, the causes may affect the infant itself after birth, in which case the mother may or may not be affected. Thus the infant dies, not because the disease has been imparted, as in the first case, but rather because childbed fever originates in the infant itself. If the mother imparts childbed fever to the infant during intrauterine life, then the difference in infant mortality between the two clinics cannot be explained by the accepted etiology, because this etiology inadequately explains the origin of the disease in mothers. If the cause of childbed fever operates directly on the infant independently of the mother, then it is still impossible for the accepted etiology to explain the difference in infant mortality rates. [Given the accepted theories], one would expect the mortality in the second clinic to have been either equal to or greater than that of the first. *[42]* Of course, many of the causal factors that purportedly explain childbed fever among maternity patients are simply impossible with regard to infants—infants would not, in all probability, fear the evil reputation of the first clinic, their modesty would not be offended by having been delivered in the presence of men, etc.

Childbed fever is defined as a disease characteristic of and limited to maternity patients, for whose origin the puerperal state and a specific causal moment are necessary.[9] Thus when this cause operates on a person who is predisposed by the puerperal state, childbed fever results. However, if this same cause operates on persons who are not puerperae, some disease other than puerperal fever is generated. For example, some believe that maternity patients in the first clinic, knowing of the countless deaths occurring there each year, are so frightened that they contract the disease. Thus the disposing factor is the puerperal state, and the precipitating factor is fear of death. We can assume that many soldiers engaged in murderous battle must also fear death. How-

---

9. Among Semmelweis's contemporaries the causal explanation of a specific instance of some disease was usually divided into predisposing and exciting factors. Different diseases were believed to result from the operation of a constant, exciting cause if the persons on whom that cause operated had been differently predisposed. In this and the following two paragraphs Semmelweis is subjecting this doctrine to ironic criticism.

ever, these soldiers do not contract childbed fever, because they are not puerperae and so they lack the disposing factor.

[43] If an individual is openly examined for the instruction of males, her modesty is offended and, because she is predisposed by the puerperal state, she contracts childbed fever. But female modesty can be offended in many ways, and if the offended young woman is not in the puerperal state, she does not contract childbed fever because she is not predisposed. Something else occurs; for example, she may swoon. Chilling brings childbed fever in puerperae, but in other persons it causes rheumatic fever. In puerperae, mistakes in diet induce childbed fever. In others, similar mistakes cause only gastric fever.

Becoming convinced that childbed fever is not restricted to puerperae and that it can begin during birth or even in pregnancy, one may ignore the puerperal state and focus on the unique composition of the blood during pregnancy. But even if we adopt such an approach, what predisposes the newborn to puerperal disease? Surely not the puerperal condition of their genitals. Do both male and female have the blood composition uniquely characteristic of pregnancy? The occurrence of childbed fever among the newborn shows that the very conception of puerperal fever is erroneous.

Because Vienna is so large, women in labor often deliver on the street, on the glacis,[10] or in front of the gates of houses before they can reach the hospital. It is then necessary for the woman, carrying her infant in her skirts, and often in very bad weather, to walk to the maternity hospital. *[44]* Such births are referred to as street births. Admission to the maternity clinic and to the foundling home is gratis, on the condition that those admitted be available for open instructional purposes, and that those fit to do so serve as wet nurses for the foundling home. Infants not born in the maternity clinic are not admitted gratis to the foundling home because their mothers have not been available for in-

10. While Semmelweis was in the first clinic, Vienna was still surrounded by medieval fortifications. The glacis was a broad earthwork that sloped away from the city and that constituted part of the fortifications. Between 1857 and 1865 the city walls were demolished and were replaced by gardens, boulevards, and public buildings.

struction. However, in order that those who had the intention of delivering in the maternity hospital but who delivered on the way would not innocently lose their privilege, street births were counted as hospital deliveries. This, however, led to the following abuse: women in somewhat better circumstances, seeking to avoid the unpleasantness of open examination without losing the benefit of having their infants accepted gratis to the foundling home, would be delivered by midwives in the city and then be taken quickly by coach to the clinic where they claimed that the birth had occurred unexpectedly while they were on their way to the clinic. If the child had not been christened and if the umbilical cord was still fresh, these cases were treated as street births, and the mother received charity exactly like those who delivered at the hospital. The number of these cases was high; frequently in a single month between the two clinics there were as many as one hundred cases.

As I have noted, women who delivered on the street contracted childbed fever at a significantly lower rate than those who delivered in the hospital. This was in spite of the less favorable conditions in which such births took place. *[45]* Of course, in most of these cases delivery occurred in a bed with the assistance of a midwife. Moreover, after three hours our patients were obliged to walk to their beds by way of the glass-enclosed passageway. However, such inconvenience is certainly less dangerous than being delivered by a midwife, then immediately having to arise, walk down many flights of stairs to the waiting carriage, travel in all weather conditions and over horribly rough pavement to the maternity hospital, and there having to climb up another flight of stairs. For those who really gave birth on the street, the conditions would have been even more difficult.

To me, it appeared logical that patients who experienced street births would become ill at least as frequently as those who delivered in the clinic. I have already expressed my firm conviction that the deaths in the first clinic were not caused by epidemic influences but by endemic and as yet unknown factors, that is, factors whose harmful influences were limited to the first clinic. What protected those who delivered outside the clinic from these destructive unknown endemic influences? In the second clinic, the health of the patients who underwent street births was as good as in the first clinic, but there the difference was not so striking, since the health of the patients was generally much better.

This would be the place to exhibit a table showing that the mortality rate among those who delivered on the street was lower than among those who delivered in the first clinic. *[46]* While I had access to the records of the first clinic I felt that such a table was unnecessary because no one denied these facts. Thus I neglected to complete a table. Later when I was no longer assistant, these facts were denied, as was the existence of a significant difference in mortality between the clinics. Because of Table 1, however, this difference is undeniable. In 1848 Professor [Josef] Skoda[11] proposed that the faculty of the Viennese medical school nominate a commission that, among other things, would construct such a table. The proposal was adopted by a great majority, and the commission was immediately named. However, as a result of protests by the Professor of Obstetrics, higher authorities intervened and the commission was unable to begin its activity.[12]

In addition to those who delivered on the street, those who delivered prematurely also became ill much less frequently than ordinary patients. Those who delivered prematurely were not only exposed to all the same endemic influences as patients who

11. Josef Skoda (1805–81) was head of the department for thoracic diseases, and from 1846 until 1871 he was Professor of Medicine at the University of Vienna. Skoda pioneered auscultation and repercussion as diagnostic techniques, and popularized the use of the stethoscope. He supported Semmelweis at the beginning, but seems never to have accepted Semmelweis's strategy of characterizing diseases etiologically. After Semmelweis left Vienna for Budapest in 1850, Skoda apparently never again mentioned Semmelweis or his works—not even in lectures on puerperal diseases.

12. The Professor of Obstetrics was Johann Klein. The proposal was, in fact, adopted unanimously, which means that even Klein approved of having a commission investigate Semmelweis's findings. But when the commission was named, Klein was not included. Thus, he would not have been a member of the commission that was to investigate work done in his own clinic. This may have led him to protest to the ministry. Erna Lesky, *Ignaz Philipp Semmelweis und die Wiener medizinische Schule* (Vienna: Hermann Böhlaus, 1964), pp. 11–35.

went full-term, they also suffered the additional harm of whatever caused the premature delivery. Under these circumstances, how could their superior health be explained? One explanation was that the earlier the birth, the less developed the puerperal condition and therefore the smaller the predisposition for the disease. Yet puerperal fever can begin during birth or even during pregnancy; indeed, even at these times it can be fatal. The better health of patients who delivered prematurely in the second clinic conformed to the general superior health of full-term patients in the clinic.

[47] Patients often became ill sporadically. One diseased patient would be surrounded by healthy patients. But very often whole rows would become ill without a single patient in the row remaining healthy. The beds in the maternity wards were arranged along the length of the rooms and were separated by equal spaces. Depending on their location, rooms in the clinic extended either north-south or east-west. If patients in beds along the north walls became ill we were often inclined to regard chilling as a significant factor. However, on the next occasion those along the south wall would become ill. Many times those on the east and west walls would become diseased. Often the disease spread from one side to the other, so that no one location seemed better or worse. How could these events be explained, given that the same patterns did not appear in the second clinic where one encountered the disease only sporadically?

It was my firm conviction that childbed fever was not contagious and did not spread from bed to bed. Later we will consider the proof for this conviction.[13] For now, it is sufficient to note that the disease appeared only sporadically in the second clinic. If childbed fever were contagious, from the sporadic cases whole rows would become ill as the disease spread from bed to bed.

[48] The authorities did not remain indifferent to the disturbing difference in mortality rates between the two clinics. Commissions repeatedly investigated and conducted hearings to determine the cause of the difference, and to decide whether it was possible to save a larger number of those patients who became

13. See below, pp. 117f., 147f.; German edition, pp. 107f., 193f.

ill. To achieve this last goal, from time to time all the diseased patients were transferred to the general hospital. But in spite of the change in physicians, rooms, and medical procedures, etc., the patients died almost without exception. The commissions would conclude that the cause of the great mortality rate was one or another or several of the endemic factors previously discussed. Various suitable measures were adopted, but none succeeded in bringing the death rate within the limits set by the second clinic. The failure of these measures proved that the factors identified were not, in fact, the relevant causes.

Toward the end of 1846 an opinion prevailed in one commission that the disease originated from damage to the birth canal inflicted during the examinations that were part of the instructional process. However, since similar examinations were part of the instruction of midwives, the increased incidence of disease in the clinic for physicians was made intelligible by assuming that male students, particularly foreigners, were too rough in their examinations. *[49]* As a result of this opinion the number of students was reduced from forty-two to twenty. Foreigners were almost entirely excluded, and examinations were reduced to a minimum. The mortality rate did decline significantly in December 1846, and in January, February, and March of 1847. But in spite of these measures, fifty-seven patients died in April and thirty-six more in May. This demonstrated to everyone that the view was groundless. To further the reader's understanding, Table 5 shows the mortality figures for 1846 and for the first five months of 1847. *[50]* We will come back later to the fact that from December 1846 through March 1847 the mortality rate declined, and that it climbed back up again in April and May 1847.[14]

Recommendations based on studies of the cause of the great mortality in the first clinic all involved one inexplicable contradiction: given the concept of an epidemic, and given that the commissions did not have the power to change the atmospheric-cosmic-terrestrial conditions of Vienna, they should have concluded that no remedies were possible. But they did not draw this conclusion, even though they considered the deaths an epidemic. What does one do to shorten the duration or to prevent

14. See below, pp. 101–5; German edition, pp. 71–75.

	Births	Deaths	Rate
1846			
Jan.	336	45	13.39
Feb.	293	53	18.08
Mar.	311	48	15.43
Apr.	253	48	18.97
May	305	41	13.44
Jun.	266	27	10.15
Jul.	252	33	13.10
Aug.	216	39	18.05
Sept.	271	39	14.39
Oct.	254	38	14.98
Nov.	297	32	10.77
Dec.	298	16	5.37
1847			
Jan.	311	10	3.21
Feb.	912	6	1.92
Mar.	305	11	3.60
Apr.	312	57	18.27
May	294	36	12.24

the recurrence of a cholera epidemic? They attributed the disease to one or more of the previously identified endemic causes. They did not, however, identify it as an endemic disease, which would have been appropriate, but rather as an epidemic. In general, the unfortunate confusion in the concepts of epidemic and endemic disease delayed discovery of the true cause of childbed fever.

In classifying puerperal disease as epidemic or endemic, one must disregard entirely the number of patients who become ill or die. The cause of the illness or death determines whether the disease is epidemic or endemic. Epidemic puerperal fever is induced by atmospheric-cosmic-terrestrial influences; the concept of an epidemic does not stipulate whether one or one hundred persons become ill. *[51]* If puerperal fever is caused by endemic factors—that is, by factors whose operation is limited to a specific location—then puerperal fever is endemic, and it is immaterial whether one or one hundred individuals become ill. This follows from the concepts of epidemic and endemic disease. In classifying the disease one way or the other, however, the commissions did not consider the purported cause but only the number of cases. Because many patients became ill and died, it was identified as an epidemic.

I was convinced that the greater mortality rate at the first clinic was due to an endemic but as yet unknown cause. That the newborn, whether female or male, also contracted childbed fever convinced me that the disease was misconceived. I was aware of many facts for which I had no explanation. Delivery with prolonged dilation almost inevitably led to death. Patients who delivered prematurely or on the street almost never became ill, and this contradicted my conviction that the deaths were due to endemic causes. The disease appeared sequentially among patients in the first clinic. Patients in the second clinic were healthier, although individuals working there were no more skillful or conscientious in their duties. The disrespect displayed by the employees toward the personnel of the first clinic made me so miserable that life seemed worthless. *[52]* Everything was in question; everything seemed inexplicable; everything was doubtful. Only the large number of deaths was an unquestionable reality.

The reader can appreciate my perplexity during my first period of service when I, like a drowning person grasping at a straw, discontinued supine deliveries, which had been customary in the first clinic, in favor of deliveries from a lateral position. I did this for no other reason than that the latter were customary in the second clinic. I did not believe that the supine position was so detrimental that additional deaths could be attributed to its use. But in the second clinic deliveries were performed from a lateral position and the patients were healthier. Consequently, we also delivered from the lateral position, so that everything would be exactly as in the second clinic.

I spent the winter of 1846–47 studying English. I did this because my predecessor, Dr. Breit, resumed the position of assistant, and I wanted to spend time in the large Dublin maternity hospital. Then, at the end of February 1847, Dr. Breit was named Professor of Obstetrics at the medical school in Tübingen. I changed my travel plans and, in the company of two friends, departed for Venice on 2 March 1847. I hoped the Venetian art treasures would revive my mind and spirits, which had been so seriously affected by my experiences in the maternity hospital.

On 20 March of the same year, a few hours after returning to Vienna, I resumed, with rejuvenated vigor, the position of assistant in the first clinic. I was immediately overwhelmed by the sad news that Professor [Jakob] Kolletschka, whom I greatly admired, had died in the interim.

[53] The case history went as follows: Kolletschka, Professor of Forensic Medicine, often conducted autopsies for legal purposes in the company of students. During one such exercise, his finger was pricked by a student with the same knife that was being used in the autopsy. I do not recall which finger was cut. Professor Kolletschka contracted lymphangitis and phlebitis [inflammation of the lymphatic vessels and of the veins respectively] in the upper extremity. Then, while I was still in Venice, he died of bilateral pleurisy, pericarditis, peritonitis, and meningitis [inflammation of the membranes of the lungs and thoracic cavity, of the fibroserous sac surrounding the heart, of the membranes of the abdomen and pelvic cavity, and of the membranes surrounding the brain, respectively]. A few days before he died,

a metastasis also formed in one eye. I was still animated by the art treasures of Venice, but the news of Kolletschka's death agitated me still more. In this excited condition I could see clearly that the disease from which Kolletschka died was identical to that from which so many hundred maternity patients had also died. The maternity patients also had lymphangitis, peritonitis, pericarditis, pleurisy, and meningitis, and metastases also formed in many of them. Day and night I was haunted by the image of Kolletschka's disease and was forced to recognize, ever more decisively, that the disease from which Kolletschka died was identical to that from which so many maternity patients died.

Earlier, I pointed out that autopsies of the newborn disclosed results identical to those obtained in autopsies of patients dying from childbed fever. I concluded that the newborn died of childbed fever, or in other words, that they died from the same disease as the maternity patients. Since the identical results were found in Kolletschka's autopsy, the inference that Kolletschka died from the same disease was confirmed. [54] The exciting cause of Professor Kolletschka's death was known; it was the wound by the autopsy knife that had been contaminated by cadaverous particles. Not the wound, but contamination of the wound by the cadaverous particles caused his death. Kolletschka was not the first to have died in this way. I was forced to admit that if his disease was identical with the disease that killed so many maternity patients, then it must have originated from the same cause that brought it on in Kolletschka. In Kolletschka, the specific causal factor was the cadaverous particles that were introduced into his vascular system. I was compelled to ask whether cadaverous particles had been introduced into the vascular systems of those patients whom I had seen die of this identical disease. I was forced to answer affirmatively.

Because of the anatomical orientation of the Viennese medical school, professors, assistants, and students have frequent opportunity to contact cadavers. Ordinary washing with soap is not sufficient to remove all adhering cadaverous particles. This is proven by the cadaverous smell that the hands retain for a longer or shorter time. In the examination of pregnant or delivering maternity patients, the hands, contaminated with cadaverous particles, are brought into contact with the genitals of these individuals, creating the possibility of resorption. With resorption, the cadaverous particles are introduced into the vascular system of the patient. *[55]* In this way, maternity patients contract the same disease that was found in Kolletschka.

Suppose cadaverous particles adhering to hands cause the same disease among maternity patients that cadaverous particles adhering to the knife caused in Kolletschka. Then if those particles are destroyed chemically, so that in examinations patients are touched by fingers but not by cadaverous particles, the disease must be reduced. This seemed all the more likely, since I knew that when decomposing organic material is brought into contact with living organisms it may bring on decomposition.

To destroy cadaverous matter adhering to hands I used *chlorina liquida.* This practice began in the middle of May 1847; I no longer remember the specific day. Both the students and I were required to wash before examinations. After a time I ceased to use *chlorina liquida* because of its high price, and I adopted the less expensive chlorinated lime. In May 1847, during the second half of which chlorine washings were first introduced, 36 patients died—this was 12.24 percent of 294 deliveries. In the remaining seven months of 1847, the mortality rate was below that of the patients in the second clinic (see Table 6).

[56] In these seven months, of the 1,841 maternity patients cared for, 56 died (3.04 percent). In 1846, before washing with chlorine was introduced, of 4,010 patients cared for in the first clinic, 459 died (11.4 percent). In the second clinic in 1846, of 3,754 patients, 105 died (2.7 percent). In 1847, when in approximately the middle of May I instituted washing with chlorine, in the first clinic of 3,490 patients, 176 died (5 percent). In the second clinic of 3,306 patients, 32 died (0.9 percent). In 1848, chlorine washings were employed throughout the year and of 3,556 patients, 45 died (1.27 percent). In the second clinic in the year 1848, of 3,219 patients 43 died (1.33 percent). The mortality rates for the individual months of 1848 are shown in Table 7.

[57] In March and August 1848 not a single patient died. In January 1849, of 403 births 9 died (2.23 percent). In February, of 389 births 12 died (3.08 percent). March had 406 births, and

[56] TABLE 6

	Births	Deaths	Rate
1847			
Jun.	268	6	2.38
Jul.	250	3	1.20
Aug.	264	5	1.89
Sept.	262	12	5.23
Oct.	278	11	3.95
Nov.	246	11	4.47
Dec.	273	8	2.93
Total	1,841	56	
Avg.			3.04

[57] TABLE 7

1848	Births	Deaths	Rate
Jan.	283	10	3.53
Feb.	291	2	0.68
Mar.	276	0	0.00
Apr.	305	2	0.65
May	313	3	0.99
Jun.	264	3	1.13
Jul.	269	1	0.37
Aug.	261	0	0.00
Sept.	312	3	0.96
Oct.	299	7	2.34
Nov.	310	9	2.90
Dec.	373	5	1.34
Total	3,556	45	
Avg.			1.27

there were 20 deaths (4.9 percent). On 20 March Dr. Carl Braun[15] succeeded me as assistant.

As mentioned, the commissions identified various endemic factors as causes of the greater mortality rate in the first clinic. Accordingly, various measures were instituted, but none brought the mortality rate within that of the second clinic. *[58]* Thus one could infer that the factors identified by the commissions were not causally responsible for the greater mortality in the first clinic. I assumed that the cause of the greater mortality rate was cadaverous particles adhering to the hands of examining obstetricians. I removed this cause by chlorine washings. Consequently, mortality in the first clinic fell below that of the second. I therefore concluded that cadaverous matter adhering to the hands of the physicians was, in reality, the cause of the increased mortality rate in the first clinic. Since the chlorine washings were instituted with such dramatic success, not even the smallest additional changes in the procedures of the first clinic were adopted to which the decline in mortality could be even partially attributed. The instruction system for midwives is so instituted that pupils and instructors have less frequent occasion to contaminate their hands with cadaverous matter than is the case in the first clinic. Thus, the unknown endemic cause of the horrible devastations in the first clinic was the cadaverous particles adhering to the hands of the examiners.

In order to destroy the cadaverous material, it was necessary that every examiner wash in chlorinated lime upon entry into the labor room. *[59]* Because students in the labor room had no opportunity to contaminate their hands anew, I believed one washing was sufficient. Because of the large number who gave birth each year in the first clinic, patients were seldom alone in the labor room; as a rule several were there simultaneously. For purposes of instruction, those in labor were arranged and ex-

15. Carl Braun (1822–91) was Klein's assistant from 1849 until 1853. He succeeded Klein as Professor of Obstetrics at the University of Vienna and became Rector of the University. Braun was consistently hostile to Semmelweis; he was not conscientious in using the prophylactic measures necessary to prevent childbed fever, and he did not accept Semmelweis's etiological characterization of the disease.

amined sequentially. I regarded it as sufficient that after each examination the hands were washed with soap and water only. Within the labor room, it seemed unnecessary for the hands to be washed with chlorine water between examinations. Once the hands had been cleaned of cadaverous particles, they could not become contaminated again.

In October 1847, a patient was admitted with discharging medullary carcinoma [cancer of the innermost part] of the uterus. She was assigned the bed at which the rounds were always initiated. After examining this patient, those conducting the examination washed their hands with soap only. The consequence was that of twelve patients then delivering, eleven died. The ichor from the discharging medullary carcinoma was not destroyed by soap and water. In the examinations, ichor was transferred to the remaining patients, and so childbed fever multiplied. Thus, childbed fever is caused not only by cadaverous particles adhering to hands but also by ichor from living organisms. It is necessary to clean the hands with chlorine water, not only when one has been handling cadavers but also after examinations in which the hands could become contaminated with ichor. [60] This rule, originating from this tragic experience, was followed thereafter. Childbed fever was no longer spread by ichor carried on the hands of examiners from one patient to another.

A new tragic experience persuaded me that air could also carry decaying organic matter. In November of the same year, an individual was admitted with a discharging carious left knee. In the genital region this person was completely healthy. Thus the examiners' hands presented no danger to the other patients. But the ichorous exhalations of the carious knee completely saturated the air of her ward. In this way the other patients were exposed and nearly all the patients in that room died. The reports of the first clinic indicate that eleven patients died in November and eight more in December. These deaths were largely due to ichorous exhalations from this individual. The ichorous particles that saturated the air of the maternity ward penetrated the uteruses already lacerated in the birth process. The particles were resorbed, and childbed fever resulted. Thereafter, such individuals were isolated to prevent similar tragedies.

[61] The maternity hospital in Vienna was opened on 16 August 1784. In the eighteenth century and in the early decades of the nineteenth century, medicine was concerned with theoretical speculation, and the anatomical foundations were neglected. Thus in 1822, of 3,066 patients only 26 died (.84 percent). In 1841, after the Viennese medical school adopted an anatomical orientation, of 3,036 patients 237 died (7.7 percent). In 1843 of 3,060 patients 274 died (8.9 percent). In 1827, of 3,294 patients 55 died (1.66 percent). In 1842 of 3,287 patients 518 died (15.8 percent).[16] From 1784 until 1823, over a period of twenty-five years, less than 1 percent of the patients cared for in the maternity hospital died. This is shown in Table 8.

[62–63] This table provides unchallengeable proof for my opinion that childbed fever originates with the spread of animal-organic matter. At the time when the educational system limited opportunities for spreading decaying animal-organic matter, the patients cared for in the maternity hospital were much healthier.

As the Viennese medical school adopted an anatomical orientation, the health of the maternity patients worsened. When the number of births and of students became so great that one professor could not supervise the births and give instruction, the maternity hospital was divided into two clinics. At that time the same number of male and female students were assigned to each clinic. On 10 October 1840, by imperial decree, all males were assigned to the first clinic and all female students to the second. I am not able to say in which year the maternity hospital was divided. Colleagues who taught obstetrics in the second clinic when male students were still admitted report that there was, at that time, no significant difference in mortality between the clinics. The consistently unfavorable health of patients in the first clinic dates from 1840, when all male students were assigned to the first clinic and all female students to the second. After what has been reported, it would be superfluous to explain these facts further.

[64] Table 1 indicates the difference in mortality rates between

16. The figures for 1841, 1842, and 1843 are for the first clinic only, see Table 1.

the patients of the two clinics after the first was devoted exclusively to training obstetricians and the second to training midwives. This would be the place to provide a similar table for the years during which female and male students were divided equally between both clinics. It would show that during this time the mortality rate was not consistently larger in the first clinic. However, I do not have access to the necessary data. The reports were prepared in triplicate in both clinics. One copy remained in the institution; one copy was sent to the governmental administration. Those who now have these reports would do a service to science if they would release them to the public.[17] I possess the reports of both clinics only for 1840, when the male and female students were separated, and for the preceding year (see Table 9). The variation in mortality for both clinics can be traced to the activities of those in the process of becoming physicians. *[65]* I was obstructed in disclosing this information because at the time it was construed as a basis for personal denunciation.

Professor Skoda assigned various responsibilities to the above-mentioned commission of the Viennese medical college. Among these were the construction of a table showing, as far as the data was available, the number of deliveries and of deaths month by month, and a list of the assistants and students in the sequential order in which they served and practiced in the maternity hospital. Professor [Karl] Rokitansky[18] has directed the pathological-anatomical division since 1828. From his recollections, and from autopsy reports, and with the help of other physicians and of the assistants and students who participated in the examination of

17. On page 130; German edition, page 139, Semmelweis reports that he has just obtained this information and proceeds to give the table that he here omits. He refers back to this page and apologizes for not including the information where it was first needed. The figures for 1839 and 1840 were made public in Carl Haller's report on the operation of the Vienna General Hospital published in the *Zeitschrift der k. k. Gesellschaft der Ärzte zu Wien*, 5, no. 2 (1849): 535–46.

18. Karl Rokitansky (1804–1878) was Professor of Pathological Anatomy at the University of Vienna from 1844 until 1875 and was Rector of the University in 1853. He was one of the outstanding anatomists of the century—he is said to have performed more than 30,000 autopsies. Rokitansky also supported Semmelweis against the older members of the faculty until Semmelweis left Vienna in 1850.

[62] TABLE 8

	Births	Deaths	Rate	Year	Births	Deaths	Rate
1784	284	6	2.11	1817	2,735	25	0.91
1785	899	13	1.44	1818	2,568	56	2.18
1786	1,151	5	0.43	1819	3,089	154	4.98
1787	1,407	5	0.35	1820	2,998	75	2.50
1788	1,425	5	0.35	1821	3,294	55	1.66
1789	1,246	7	0.56	1822	3,066	26	0.84
1790	1,326	10	0.75	1823	2,872	214	7.45
1791	1,395	8	0.57	1824	2,911	144	4.94
1792	1,574	14	0.89	1825	2,594	229	4.82
1793	1,684	44	2.61	1826	2,359	192	8.12
1794	1,768	7	0.39	1827	2,367	51	2.15
1795	1,798	38	2.11	1828	2,833	101	3.56
1796	1,904	22	1.16	1829	3,012	140	4.64
1797	2,012	5	0.24	1830	2,797	111	3.97
1798	2,046	5	0.24	1831	3,353	222	6.62

Year				Year			
1799	2,067	20	0.96	1832	3,331	105	3.15
1800	2,070	41	1.98	1833	3,907	205	5.25
1801	2,106	17	0.80	1834	4,218	355	8.41
1802	2,346	9	0.38	1835	4,040	227	5.61
1803	2,215	16	0.72	1836	4,144	331	7.98
1804	2,022	8	0.39	1837	4,363	375	8.59
1805	2,112	9	0.40	1838	4,560	179	3.92
1806	1,875	13	0.73	1839	4,992	248	4.96
1807	925	6	0.64	1840	5,166	328	6.44
1808	855	7	0.81	1841	5,454	330	6.05
1809	912	13	1.42	1842	6,024	730	12.11
1810	744	6	0.80	1843	5,914	457	7.72
1811	1,050	20	1.90	1844	6,244	336	5.38
1812	1,419	9	0.63	1845	6,756	313	4.63
1813	1,945	21	1.08	1846	7,027	567	8.06
1814	2,062	66	3.20	1847	7,039	210	2.98
1815	2,591	19	0.73	1848	7,095	91	1.28
1816	2,410	12	0.49				

[64] TABLE 9

	First Clinic			Second Clinic		
	Births	Deaths	Rate	Births	Deaths	Rate
1839	2,781	151	5.4	2,010	91	4.5
1840	2,889	267	9.5	2,073	55	2.6

corpses, it would be possible to determine whether the number of diseased patients corresponded to the activities of assistants and students in the autopsy room. As mentioned above, higher authorities prevented the commission from carrying out this assignment.

In consequence of my conviction I must affirm that only God knows the number of patients who went prematurely to their graves because of me. I have examined corpses to an extent equaled by few other obstetricians. If I say this also of another physician, my intention is only to bring to consciousness a truth that, to humanity's great misfortune, has remained unknown through so many centuries. No matter how painful and oppressive such a recognition may be, the remedy does not lie in suppression. If the misfortune is not to persist forever, then this truth must be made known to everyone concerned.

[66] After it was realized that the additional deaths in the first clinic were explained by cadaverous and ichorous particles on the examiners' contaminated hands, various unexplained phenomena could be accounted for quite naturally. In the morning hours the professor and the students made general rounds; in the afternoons the assistant and the students made rounds. As part of their instruction, the students examined all patients who were pregnant or in labor. The assistant was also obliged, before the morning visit of the professor, to examine those in labor and to report on them to the professor. Between these visits the assistant and the students would assume responsibility for necessary examinations. When, therefore, dilation extended over a long period and the patient spent one or more days in the labor room, she was certain to be examined repeatedly by persons whose hands were contaminated with cadaverous and ichorous particles. In this way childbed fever was induced, and as I have

mentioned, these individuals died almost without exception. Once the chlorine washings were adopted and the patients were examined only by persons with clean hands, patients with extended periods of dilation stopped dying, and extended labor was no more dangerous than in the second clinic.

In order to make my next point intelligible, I must partially explain how I conceive of childbed fever. For now it is sufficient to observe that foul animal-organic particles are resorbed, and that in consequence of this resorption, disintegration of the blood [*Blutentmischung*] sets in. *[67]* We have already noted that those with extended periods of dilation contracted rapidly developing childbed fever either during birth or directly thereafter. In other words, the resorption of foul animal-organic particles and the resulting disintegration of the mother's blood occurred at a time when the fetal blood was in organic exchange through the placenta with the blood of the mother. In this way, blood disintegration, from which the mother was suffering, was transmitted to the child. In consequence the newborn, whether female or male, died from a disease identical to that of the mother and in numbers equal to the mothers. Childbed fever originates in the mother because foul animal-organic matter is resorbed and leads to blood disintegration. In the infant the situation is somewhat different. The fetus, as yet unborn and in the birth canal, does not resorb foul animal-organic matter when it is touched by the examiner's contaminated fingers, but only when its blood is organically mixed with the mother's blood that has already become contaminated. This explains why an infant never dies of childbed fever while the mother remains healthy; childbed fever does not arise in the newborn through direct resorption. *[68]* Both become ill while the child and mother are in organic interchange through the placenta and when the blood of the mother has disintegrated through the resorption of foul animal-organic matter. The mother can become ill while the child remains healthy if the organic interchange between them is ended by the birth process before disintegration of the mother's blood has begun.

As I have said, cadaverous particles adhering to the hands were destroyed by chlorine washings. In this way, the incidence of disease among maternity patients was brought within the limits set in the second clinic. Chlorine washings had the same effect on the incidence of disease among the newborn. Healthy mothers could no longer impart childbed fever to their infants.

In 1846, without chlorine washing, of 3,533 infants in the first clinic, 235 died (6 percent). In the second clinic, of 3,398 infants 86 died (2.5 percent). In 1847, during the last seven months of which we washed with chlorine, of 3,322 infants 167 died (5.02 percent). In the second clinic, of 3,139 infants 90 died (2.8 percent). In 1848, when chlorine washings were practiced during the entire year, of 3,496 infants 147 died in the first clinic (4.2 percent). In the second clinic 100 infants died, out of 3,089 (3.2 percent). *[69]* These infant deaths were not from childbed fever.

If a mother died before her child, or if a mother, for whatever reason, could not nurse her child, the child was taken to the foundling home. In the foundling home, many nursing infants died of childbed fever. After the introduction of chlorine washings, nursing infants in the foundling home ceased to die of childbed fever. Dr. [Alois] Bednar, then head physician of the Imperial Foundling Home in Vienna, wrote: "Sepsis of the blood of newborns has become a great rarity. For this we must thank the consequential and most noteworthy discovery of Dr. Semmelweis, emeritus assistant of the Viennese first maternity clinic. His work fortunately explained the cause and the prevention of the formerly murderous ravages of puerperal fever."[19] Where I speak of childbed fever of the newborn, Dr. Bednar correctly speaks of sepsis of the blood; he thus remains consistent with ordinary usage.

Once the cause of the increased mortality in the first clinic was identified as cadaverous particles adhering to the hands of the examiners, it was easy to explain why women who delivered in the street had a strikingly lower mortality rate than those who delivered in the clinic. This was so because once the infant was born and the placenta separated, there was generally no longer opportunity for instruction; thus there were no examinations. A

---

19. [Alois] Bednar, *Die Krankheiten der Neugeborenen und Säuglinge vom klinischen und pathologisch-anatomischen Standpunkte bearbeitet* (Vienna: Gerold, 1850), p. 198 [author's note].

bed was assigned to such patients, and they generally left it in good health. There was no reason for their genitals to be touched by contaminated hands; therefore they did not contract childbed fever. *[70]* Also, women who delivered prematurely became ill less often because they were not examined either. The first requirement in premature births is to delay birth if possible. Consequently, these persons were not used for open instruction, and decaying organic matter was not conveyed to their genitals.

The sequential appearance of disease was also easy to explain. Because of the large number of births in the first clinic, several individuals were often in the labor room simultaneously. These persons were examined at least twice a day—during the morning rounds of the professor, and during the afternoon rounds of the assistant. Everyone in labor was examined for instruction sequentially in the order of their beds. When, therefore, the examiners' hands were contaminated with cadaverous particles, the genitals of several individuals were simultaneously brought into contact with cadaverous particles. This meant that the germ [*Keim*] for childbed fever was planted through resorption in several individuals at once. The patients were placed back in the maternity ward in the order in which they had delivered. Thus it often happened that those who were together in the labor room delivered at about the same time and thereafter remained in the same sequential order in the maternity clinic. In the labor room they were examined in rows by persons whose hands were contaminated with cadaverous particles, the germ of the future puerperal fever, and the disease occurred among them sequentially. *[71]* After chlorine washing was instituted, sequential cases of the disease ceased.

I mentioned that toward the end of 1846, because of the prevalence of childbed fever in the first clinic, yet another commission was instituted—I have no idea how many times this had already been done—in order to identify the cause of these deaths. This commission identified the cause as injury to genitals inflicted during instructional examinations. But because the same examinations were conducted for the instruction of midwives, the commission explained that male students, particularly foreigners, examined too roughly. Consequently, the number of students was reduced to a minimum. Table 5 shows how great the mortality was before this measure was adopted, how it then declined, and how, in the months of April and May, it increased again in spite of the preventive measures. I will now explain these phenomena. Before I do, however, one item must be discussed.

As an aspirant for the position of assistant in the first clinic, later as provisional assistant and then, finally, as actual assistant, it was not possible for me to study gynecology at the gynecological division of the Imperial Hospital. However, such study was highly desirable for an obstetrician. As a substitute, as soon as I had decided to devote my life to obstetrics I examined all the female corpses in the morgue of the Imperial General Hospital. From 1844 until I moved to Pest in 1850, I devoted nearly every morning before the professor's rounds in the obstetrical clinic to these studies. I very much appreciate having enjoyed the friendship of Professor Rokitansky. *[72]* Through his kindness I secured permission to dissect all female corpses, including those not already set aside for autopsy, in order to correlate the results of my examinations with autopsies.

For reasons that do not concern us here, the assistant of the first clinic seldom visited the morgue in the months of December 1846 and January, February, and March 1847. The Austrian students, whose number was reduced to eighteen, followed his example. The opportunity for them to contaminate their hands with cadaverous particles was thereby greatly reduced. Restricting examinations to the minimum also reduced the opportunity for the genitals of patients to be touched by contaminated hands. For these reasons, mortality in the first clinic was reduced during these months.

On 20 March 1847, I reassumed the position of assistant in the first clinic. Early that morning I conducted my gynecological studies in the morgue. I then went to the labor room and began to examine all the patients, as my predecessors and I were obliged to do, so that I could report on each patient during the professor's morning rounds. My hands, contaminated by cadaverous particles, were thereby brought into contact with the genitals of so many women in labor that in April, from 312 deliveries, there were 57 deaths (18.26 percent). *[73]* In May, from 294 deliveries there were 36 deaths (12.24 percent). In the middle of May, without noting the exact day, I instituted chlorine washings. Thus, the great mortality in the first clinic was not caused by injuries in rough examinations—a completely false assumption—but by contaminated fingers that contacted the genitals of the patients. During April and May, when again so many died, the clinic remained the same as in earlier months, yet the mortality rate increased significantly because I intervened, my fingers contaminated with cadaverous particles.

After chlorine washings were conducted for a longer period with such beneficial results, the number of students was again increased to forty-two. One no longer took account of whether they were Austrian or foreign. The examinations were resumed as was expedient for instruction. Nevertheless, the first clinic lost the dismal distinction of having the greater mortality rate. In December 1846 and in January, February, and March of 1847, I functioned as provisional assistant and simultaneously conducted gynecological studies in the morgue, yet in these months the mortality rate remained low. The reason is that as provisional assistant I had the right, but not the duty, to examine all patients in labor. After three years in so large a maternity hospital, it was no longer instructive for me to examine all the patients. I examined only exceptional cases—that is, I examined very seldom. When I became the actual assistant, it was my duty to conduct all examinations before the professor's morning rounds. *[74]* Thereafter, it was necessary for me to examine nearly all the women in labor for the purpose of instructing the students. This occasioned the great mortality rates in April and May of 1847.

Native students are those who completed their education at an Austrian university [*Hochschule*]. Foreign students are those who were educated elsewhere and who then did further work at the great University of Vienna. In Vienna one can meet physicians from all the countries of the civilized world. The course in practical obstetrics lasted two months. The influx of students into this, the largest maternity hospital in the world, was so great that to accept simultaneously all who sought admission would have excessively disrupted the patients. Applicants were assigned numbers, and were accepted sequentially to replace departing students, regardless of whether they were native or foreign. Each student was free to repeat the course as often as he felt it necessary for his own obstetrical training. However, in order that those who wished to repeat the course would not remain constantly enrolled, precluding others from taking it at all, it was necessary that one wait three months after completing the course before enrolling again. The commission charged the foreigners with being more dangerous than the natives because they were rough in examinations and, consequently, at any one time only two foreigners were allowed to attend the course in practical obstetrics. Everyone, even those who do not share my opinion, will agree that the commission acted groundlessly in imputing guilt to the foreigners. In fact, I alone held that foreigners *were* more dangerous than natives, but not because they examined more roughly. *[75]* The reason that foreigners were more dangerous than natives lies in the following considerations.

Foreigners come to Vienna to perfect medical training already begun in their own universities. They visit pathological and forensic autopsies in the general hospital. They take courses in pathological anatomy, in surgery, obstetrics, microscopic surgery of cadavers, they visit the medical and surgical wards of the hospital, etc. In a word, they utilize their time as efficiently and educationally as possible. They have, therefore, many opportunities for their hands to become contaminated with foul animal-organic matter. Thus, it is no wonder that foreigners, busy in the maternity hospital at the same time, are more dangerous for patients. Natives take the course in practical obstetrics after completing two difficult examinations in order to attain the degree of Doctor of Medicine. The law stipulates that the minimum preparation time for these examinations is six months. Thus the natives have already toiled excessively before they are admitted into the maternity hospital, and they regard the time there as a rest. While enrolled in practical obstetrics, natives do not concern themselves with other activities that would contaminate their hands. Indeed, while working at the maternity hospital,

they concern themselves even less with other aspects of medicine because, after completing the course, they can perfect their
knowledge of medicine to the highest possible degree. Since the
foreigners are generally able to remain in Vienna only a few
months, they are compelled to work simultaneously in more
than one aspect of medicine. Even so, one cannot impute guilt
to the foreigners any more than to me or to all the others who
undertook examinations with contaminated hands. None of us
knew that we were causing the numerous deaths.

[76] In order to confirm my views directly, I felt it was necessary to conduct animal experiments. With my friend, Dr.
[George Maria] Lautner, assistant to Professor Rokitansky, I carried out experiments on rabbits. [Semmelweis devotes several
pages to technical descriptions of the experiments, we continue
with his summary.] *[77–80]* . . . It is hardly necessary to mention that the changes discovered in dissecting the rabbits are the
same as those found in human bodies in consequence of puerperal diseases and, in general, in consequence of pyemia.

At the end of my two-year period of service I requested an
extension of two additional years as had been awarded to Dr.
Breit, my predecessor. Such an extension would have enabled
me to further support my opinions on the origin of childbed
fever; these opinions had occasioned numerous denials. My request was not granted, although at the same time my colleague
in the second clinic [Franz Zipfl] was awarded a similar opportunity. *[81]* Indeed, my successor [Carl Braun] was also given a
two-year extension of his period of service.

On 20 March 1849, after being released from the position of
assistant, I petitioned to be made private docent of obstetrics.[20]
My attempt met with no success. After a second petition and an
eight-month wait, on 10 October 1850 I was named private docent of theoretical obstetrics, but I was limited to demonstrating
and practicing on manikins. Such a limited docentship was of
no use to me. While the law required equally encompassing in-

---

20. A private docent was a private lecturer or teacher who taught university
students, but who was inferior in rank to a professor. A docent was often paid
directly by the students with whom he worked.

struction for licensing a docent as for a professor, professors were permitted to demonstrate and to practice on cadavers. In October 1850, therefore, I returned to my native city of Pest.

One of the first evenings after I returned to Pest was spent in the company of a large number of physicians. Because of my presence, the conversation turned to childbed fever. Objections to my opinions regarding the origin of the disease were expressed. It was claimed that at that very time in the maternity ward of St. Rochus Hospital in Pest an epidemic of childbed fever was raging. Since the hospital was not a teaching institution, however, no students were examining patients with hands contaminated by decaying animal-organic matter.

On the following morning, in order to convince myself, I visited the maternity hospital. There I found a corpse, not yet removed, of a person who had just died of puerperal fever, another patient in severe agony, and four others seriously ill with the disease. The other persons present were not maternity patients but suffered from various disorders. *[82]* Thus the unhealthy condition of the maternity patients was clearly established, but this did not contradict but rather confirmed my opinion on the origin of childbed fever. Closer inspection disclosed that the obstetrical ward was not independent but was assigned to a surgical ward. The head physician of obstetrics was simultaneously a head surgeon and a juridical anatomist. Moreover, lacking a coroner, the various division physicians were obliged to perform autopsies. The head physician first visited the surgical wards and then the maternity ward. Thus, while the obstetrical ward of the St. Rochus Hospital had no student examiners whose hands were contaminated with decaying animal-organic matter, the head physician and the other physicians assigned to him, having visited the surgical ward, did examine with contaminated hands.

I have shown that the great mortality in the first clinic derived from the cadaverous particles adhering to the hands of the examiners. I have shown that in October 1847, ichorous particles from a discharging medullary carcinoma of the uterus brought on childbed fever. I have also shown that in November 1847, exuded ichorous particles from a carious knee brought on the disease. At the maternity ward of St. Rochus Hospital, the causal

factor of childbed fever was the decaying animal-organic substances that are found so abundantly in a surgical ward. *[83]* It
may be necessary to say a few words about the maternity ward
in the St. Rochus Hospital.

The St. Rochus Hospital belongs to the community of Pest
and has a capacity of 600 patients, with three medical and two
surgical head physicians. As already mentioned, the maternity
ward was assigned to a head surgeon. As long as the obstetrical
clinic of the Pest medical faculty is open, the St. Rochus Hospital does not admit maternity patients. This is in order that the
clinic will not lack cases for instructional purposes. Only during
the major vacation in August and September, when the obstetrical clinic of the Pest medical faculty is closed, are maternity
patients admitted to St. Rochus Hospital. For the remaining ten
months of the year, the area in which the maternity ward is located is used as a surgical ward. During the school year, only
those women delivered who happened to go into labor while
they were in St. Rochus Hospital suffering from miscellaneous
illnesses. The obstetrical ward is located on the third floor of the
building, and consists of a labor room and two maternity rooms.
All six windows of these rooms overlook the morgue. Running
beside the building in which the morgue is located is a wide
street which partially dissipates the noxious exhalations of the
morgue.

On 20 May 1851, I assumed the position of unpaid, honorary
head physician of the obstetrical ward of the St. Rochus Hospital, thus dissolving the connection with the surgical wards. I
functioned in this capacity for six years, until June 1857. During
the school year, the location of the maternity ward became a
gynecological rather than a surgical ward. *[84]* This removed
the causal factor that had previously occasioned childbed fever,
namely the degenerating animal-organic matter from the surgical ward. Consequently, childbed fever declined significantly.

We did not ordinarily employ chlorine washings, because we
had no need to purify our hands from decaying animal-organic
material. After the few autopsies that I was obliged to perform,
I cleaned my hands with chloride of lime. In the vacation months
of the school year 1850–51, there were 121 births recorded in

the maternity ward at St. Rochus Hospital. In succeeding years there were 189, 142, 156, 199, and 126 births. By 1855–56 there had been, therefore, 933 births. From these, 24 patients died, and of these only 8 from childbed fever (.85 percent). The remaining 16 died of the various diseases for which they were being treated while pregnant. At the onset of labor they had been transferred to the maternity ward. Of the 8 patients who died of childbed fever, 1 contracted the disease as follows: because of the breech position of the fetus, the mother was examined by an assistant surgeon. And this occurred just after he had performed an autopsy on a man who died of a gangrenous leg. Thus, in the maternity clinic of the St. Rochus Hospital over a period of six years, less than 1 percent of the maternity patients died of childbed fever. Formerly each year childbed fever had claimed many lives.

[85] On 18 July 1855, I was named Professor of Theoretical and Practical Obstetrics at the University of Pest. I began my activities in the obstetrical clinic in October of the same year. The obstetrical clinic is located on the third floor of the faculty building and consists of a labor room and four maternity rooms. In order to acquaint the reader with the conditions of this clinic, I will quote part of a petition I placed with the appropriate authorities for permission to leave this highly unsanitary and inconvenient location:

> The following considerations show that the obstetrical clinic is highly unsanitary: imperial ordinances stipulate that hospitals will have 16 square yards [*vier Quadratklafter* = 4 square fathoms] for each maternity bed. Since the obstetrical clinic has twenty-six beds, this ordinance requires 416 square yards. However, the clinic has only 164 square yards. Moreover, it lacks the space that is required for a large number of students. Three rooms are so small that not even half the students can gain admission at one time. The other two rooms are barely large enough to accommodate all the students without pressing them together so much that they are immobile. The air becomes so stale that it is dangerous to the patients; every disinterested person recognizes this. [86] Three smokestacks from the chemical laboratory are in the window columns of two of the rooms. When there are fires in the corresponding hearths, the temperature in these rooms becomes un-

bearable. The obstetrical clinic is so restricted in area that no room can be reserved for those who are ill. Thus, ill patients remain scattered among the healthy, and in this way childbed fever is spread. Childbed fever is not a contagious disease, but it can, under certain circumstances, spread from one person to another.

Two of the clinic's windows open onto the northern light well and six windows onto the western. The northern shaft is 8 yards wide and a fire wall encloses it to the height of the windows of the maternity ward. The lavatories for the first three floors are in this light well. On the ground floor, next to the lavatory, is the building garbage pit. This decaying mass exudes a penetrating stench. Facilities for elementary and pathological anatomy are on the first floor. Drains from these facilities, through which all their liquid wastes are discharged, are immediately below the windows of the maternity clinic. The second floor contains the chemistry department. The morgue is between the light wells. The west light well is 2 yards wide and is enclosed by a wall 6 yards high. On the opposite side of this wall is an open field. Part of the morgue is in this shaft, and again, on the first floor are elementary and pathological anatomy, with chemistry on the second floor.

This is not the place for an exposition of the petitioner's views on childbed fever. [87] It is sufficient to note that he believes that every case of childbed fever without exception is due to the incorporation of decaying animal-organic matter. The honorable college of professors can well imagine the undesirable position of a professor of obstetrics who has this conviction and who is obliged to choose either to have the windows hermetically sealed, and so to allow his patients to grow worse by breathing air befouled by throngs of students, or to leave the windows open and to admit air saturated with corrupted organic matter.

But however dark the present situation may be, if the clinic remains in the same location it has an even more dismal future. A three-story building is to be erected on the empty lot opposite the western light well. This will totally obstruct light from the windows of the obstetrical clinic. Moreover, the exhalations from the narrow light well will no longer be dissipated over the empty lot; they will be conducted in a highly dangerous concentration from the three-story building to the windows of the obstetrical clinic.

Whether the petitioner's patients enjoy good health or die from childbed fever is not only of importance for those cared for in this clinic. The consequences of the petitioner's efforts regarding the health of his patients is of significance to all humanity.

[88] That childbed fever causes significantly more deaths in maternity hospitals than outside them is known to both physicians and laymen. In official documents, maternity hospitals are termed "deathtraps" not only by physicians but also by officials. Because childbed fever rages in the hospitals the question has been discussed repeatedly whether it would not be in the interests of humanity to close them. Only a detestable dilemma saves the maternity hospitals from destruction: if individuals deliver in a maternity hospital, childbed fever rages horribly, and many in the prime of life descend into an early grave. However, if the maternity hospitals are closed, larger numbers of women certainly remain healthy, but they become concerned about themselves and the care of their infants. Thus because of their need, the crimes of abortion, abandonment, and infanticide take place. The maternity hospitals are endured because it is believed to be better for patients to risk childbed fever inside them than to risk misery outside that may lead them to prison.

The petitioner has found the cause of childbed fever and has shown how to prevent it. The attention of advocates and opponents of these doctrines is focused on the health of the patients he treats. If their health becomes unfavorable, then the advocates of these opinions are weakened, and the opponents are strengthened in their doubts. *[89]* In this way, the spread of the petitioner's teachings will be hindered and humanity will continue to endure this plague. . . .

[90–95] [Semmelweis concludes the petition by quoting other authorities who had criticized the unsanitary conditions of the obstetrical clinic in Pest. He then notes:] In this location within ten months, 500 maternity patients are cared for, and 60 to 70 obstetricians and 180–90 midwives are trained. For obstetricians the course in practical obstetrics lasts two months; for student midwives the course lasts five months. Thus at any given time, the teacher is surrounded by at least 100 students. In the school year 1855–56, 514 maternity patients were cared for; 5 died, 2 of childbed fever (.19 percent) and 3 of other diseases. In 1856–57, 558 patients were cared for, 31 died, 16 of childbed fever (2.9 percent) and 15 of other diseases. In 1857–58, 457 patients were

cared for, 23 died, 18 of childbed fever (4.05 percent) and 5 of other diseases.

The mortality in 1856–58 resulted in an official correspondence. This is partially quoted here in order that the reader may become familiar with the cause of these deaths:

> Confidential reports have been made concerning various inappropriate circumstances in the obstetrical clinic of the Imperial University. For example, through the carelessness of the head midwife, not only is the bed linen seldom changed, but indeed, linen that is still befouled with the blood of earlier deceased patients is spread under newly admitted patients. As a result of this, mortality at the beginning of this year was so high that as many as ten patients died on a single day.
>
> *[96]* This fact is all the more striking in that during the previous year, in a period with a much lower mortality rate, this situation was noted by the Professor and a larger allocation of bed linen was sought. So much was immediately obtained that a store of bed linen was provided consisting of several hundred more sheets than were needed. Also, as requested, a quantity of bedding and personal linen was provided during the vacation. The costs were so great that they did not escape the notice of the Minister of Culture and Education.
>
> The Professor appears, therefore, to be in agreement with others who have access to the clinic in recognizing that the increase of sickness and death is not due to lack of linen, or to irregular deliveries from the laundress, but to inattention and irregularity in managing the linen.

I responded as follows:

> I am certainly in agreement with others who have access to the clinic in recognizing that the greater mortality rate of 1857–58 is not due to a lack of linen or to irregular deliveries from the laundress, but to inattention and irregularity in managing the linen. *[97]* However, an attendant, not the head midwife, was responsible. This attendant has subsequently been discharged.
>
> In 1856–57, thirty-one patients died. Sixteen of these died from childbed fever because of a lack of linen and because of irregular deliveries from the laundress. In the school year 1857–58, twenty-four patients died. Of these, eighteen died of childbed fever be-

cause of inattention and irregularity in managing the linen.

Never more than two individuals died on a given day. If one says, therefore, that in 1856–57 a much smaller mortality rate prevailed, and that at the beginning of the school year 1857–58 as many as ten patients died on a single day, one is simply not telling the truth.

Linen still befouled with the blood of dead patients was never spread under new patients. This charge must, therefore, have reference to linen that we received from the laundry in the school year 1856–57 that was supposed to have been laundered but that, in fact, was still befouled with blood and lochial discharge. I personally demonstrated, in a report, that this linen occasioned childbed fever in the clinic.[21]

From the first medical writers on, from Hippocrates until the most recent times, it was the unchallenged conviction of all physicians of all times that the horrible ravages of childbed fever among maternity patients were epidemic—that is, they were due to atmospheric influences. Influences that, notwithstanding every possible precaution of the physician, ravaged unabated and without remission. In 1847, in the great Viennese maternity hospital, I succeeded in proving that this opinion is false and that every single case of childbed fever is occasioned by infection. *[98]* In consequence of the measures suggested by my views, during twenty-one months in Vienna, six years in the St. Rochus Hospital, and one year at the clinic at Pest, I have had no epidemics. Previously all these institutions were devastated by horrible epidemics. I regard the two disastrous years that followed as unintentional, tragic, but direct proof of the accuracy of the opinion published in my report.

The beneficial consequences of my opinion regarding the generation of childbed fever have been compared with those of Jenner's cowpox inoculations. I realize how presumptuous it is to assert such a thing of myself; only the fact that precisely my clinic has been accused of greater mortality forces me to make such an assertion. Given that I am not responsible for the increased mor-

---

21. The report was "A gyermekágyi láz kóroktana [The Etiology of Childbed Fever]" published in *Orvosi hetilap* 2(1858); a translation is included in Tiberius von Györy, *Semmelweis' gesammelte Werke* (Jena: Gustav Fischer, 1905), pp. 61–83. This was Semmelweis's first publication on the subject of puerperal fever. According to Györy the substance of the report was contained in lectures delivered before the Budapester königliche Ärzteverein in the spring of 1858. Ibid., p. 601.

tality at the clinic at Pest, perhaps my nine years of shining success can be seen in a more favorable light.

From this official correspondence, the reader can easily determine that mortality among maternity patients during these two
years was caused by unclean bed linen in combination with the
generally unsanitary conditions of the clinic.

The laundry is given out to a contractor who is required to
exchange the linen weekly. During the school year 1856–57, the
responsible officials felt that too much was paid for the laundry
service, and it was released to the minimum bidder. Of course
the minimum bidder does not guarantee the best work—only
the cheapest. *[99]* The price was so reduced that it was impossible, especially in winter, to furnish clean linen. Childbed fever
was caused by the use of such poorly laundered linen. After
complaints were registered, the earlier contractor was given the
laundry again at the original price and the disease became less
frequent. In the school year 1857–58 it was again unclean linen
that occasioned the greater mortality rate, but the linen was not
delivered dirty from the contractor. Rather, the attendant neglected to change the linen regularly. Blood and lochial discharge decayed to such a degree that childbed fever was again
encountered. Through thorough cleaning of the bed linen and
the dismissal of the attendant, the mortality was again reduced. . . .

[Semmelweis repeats the various ways infection can occur, as
well as certain other conclusions. The chapter ends with this
paragraph:] *[100–101]* In the school year 1857–58, the external
genitals of two patients became gangrenous. Because of a short-
age of space, they were obliged to remain among the other patients. To isolate them as much as possible, they were cared for
by two student midwives in twelve-hour shifts. These midwives had orders not to touch any other individual. Nevertheless, one of them was caught as she prepared to examine a newly
admitted patient.[22]

22. In another essay Semmelweis reports that the patient became ill from this
examination but later recovered. Györy, op. cit., note 21 above, p. 74. He also
notes that one of the attendants had previously pricked her finger with a pin.
From the gangrenous patients she contracted puerperal fever and nearly died.
See below, pp. 148–49; German edition, p. 195.

CHAPTER 2

The Concept of Childbed Fever

[102] Based on experience of over fifteen years in three different institutions, all of which were severely afflicted with childbed fever, I regard the disease, without a single exception, as a resorption fever dependent on the resorption of decaying animal-organic matter. Resorption first causes disintegration of the blood. This is followed by exudation. In the overwhelming majority of cases the decaying animal-organic matter is conveyed to the individual from external sources. These are the cases represented as epidemics of childbed fever; these are the cases that can be prevented. Occasionally, decaying animal-organic matter is generated within the attacked organism. This is self-infection and cannot always be prevented.

The source of decaying animal-organic matter can be a corpse of any age, of either sex, regardless of the preceding disease, regardless whether the corpse is a pregnant woman or not. Only the degree of decomposition of the corpse should be taken into consideration. [103] These assorted corpses are the ones which people who practiced in the first clinic examined. The source of decaying animal-organic matter can be a diseased person of any age, of either sex, regardless whether the individual suffers from childbed fever; only whether the decaying animal-organic matter is a result of the disease comes into question. In the first clinic in October 1847 childbed fever was caused by a discharging medullary carcinoma of the uterus, and in November 1847 by the exhalations of a carious knee. In the maternity ward of the St. Rochus Hospital childbed fever was caused by the ichorous products of various surgical disorders. The source of the decaying animal-organic matter is every physiological animal-organic structure that, having been withdrawn from the vital order, has reached a specific degree of decay. Not the nature of the structure but only the degree of decomposition comes into question. In the obstetrical clinic at Pest during the school years 1856–57 and 1857–58 childbed fever was caused by physiological blood and normal lochial discharge that adhered to the bed linen and began to decay.[1]

Decaying animal-organic matter is carried by examining fingers, operating hands, instruments, bed linen, the atmosphere, sponges, basins, hands of midwives and attendants. *[104]* In other words, anything that is contaminated by decaying animal-organic matter and that comes into contact with the genitals of patients.

The decaying animal-organic matter is resorbed at the inner surface of the uterus from the external orifice upward. As a result of pregnancy, this surface is denuded of its mucous membrane and is therefore unusually resorbant. The remaining undamaged parts of the genitals, which also lack a mucous membrane, do not resorb because of the thick layer of epithelium [cells joined with cementing substances that cover all the interior and exterior surfaces of the body]. When injured, each part of the genitals can become a site of resorption. Infections seldom occur during pregnancy because, since the orifice of the uterus is closed, the resorbant inner surface is inaccessible. External infection can occur during pregnancy when the orifice of the uterus is open and the resorbant inner surface is accessible. The rarity of external infections during pregnancy is also explained by the fact that even when the orifice is open, it is seldom necessary in manual examinations to touch these inner surfaces. I have neglected to record how frequently in the first clinic childbed fever occurred during pregnancy. I believe it happened approximately twenty times a year. Childbed fever always terminates pregnancy. Only one patient died of childbed fever while

---

1. In their early accounts of Semmelweis's work, both C. H. F. Routh and Josef Skoda suggested that corpses were the only source of infection that was involved in puerperal fever. Consequently, many of Semmelweis's critics attacked this indefensible position, and his views seemed to be much weaker than they really were. This misunderstanding certainly delayed comprehension and adoption of Semmelweis's prophylactic measures. In his book Semmelweis continually stresses the other sources of contamination.

still pregnant; she was delivered by me, postmortem, by Caesarean section, in order to save the child.

[105] Infection occurs most often during dilation. Not only is
the inner surface of the uterus accessible at that time but it is also
frequently necessary to penetrate the uterus in manual examination to determine the location and position of the fetus. Thus,
before chlorine washings, almost every patient whose period of
dilation was extended died of childbed fever. During delivery
the body of the fetus, as it pushes down, renders the inner surface of the uterus inaccessible. During delivery, therefore, infection seldom occurs. Immediately after birth and thereafter, the
inner surface of the uterus is again accessible, and during this
period infection occurs, especially when air saturated with decaying animal-organic matter penetrates the genitals. In November 1847, air in the maternity rooms of the first clinic became permeated with the exudations of a carious knee. This air
penetrated the lacerated genitals of the patients and caused childbed
fever. After birth, infection can also occur when the genitals,
injured by the passage of the fetus, are brought into contact with
bed linen that is contaminated with decaying animal-organic
matter. During the school years 1856–57 and 1857–58 childbed
fever was caused by unclean linen at the obstetrical clinic in Pest.

[106] In rare cases, decaying animal-organic matter originates
inside the affected person. This occurs when organic matter that
should be discharged during delivery begins to decay before being
discharged. In being resorbed, it causes childbed fever by self-
infection. The organic matter can be lochia, decidual remnants,
clotted blood that is retained in the uterus, etc. Alternatively, the
decaying animal-organic matter can be a product of pathological
processes. For example, as a result of a difficult operation with
forceps, portions of the genitals may be crushed and become
gangrenous. Upon resorption, the gangrenous particles cause
childbed fever by self-infection.

Suppose we explain childbed fever as a fever of resorption in
which the introduction of decaying animal-organic matter leads
to disintegration of the blood and to exudation. Then childbed
fever is not a disease unique to and appearing only in the newly
delivered, because as a result of resorption the disease may arise

during pregnancy or when giving birth. The disease can be conveyed to infants, whether male or female. In consequence of resorption of decaying matter it can also be found among anatomists, surgeons, in operative cases in surgical wards, etc. Kolletschka also had this disease. Thus childbed fever is not a species of disease; rather it is a type of pyemia.

Various concepts are associated with the expression 'pyemia' and it is necessary, therefore, to explain that I understand this term as referring to disintegration of the blood through decaying animal-organic matter. *[107]* One type of pyemia I call childbed fever, because in pyemia of maternity patients one finds phenomena in the genital region that are not found in other people. Anatomists and surgeons who die of pyemia do not have endometritis [serious infection of the mucous membrane of the uterus], etc.

Childbed fever is not a contagious disease. A contagious disease is one that produces the contagion by which the disease is spread. This contagion brings about only the same disease in other individuals. Smallpox is a contagious disease because smallpox generates the contagion that causes smallpox in others. Smallpox causes only smallpox and no other disease. Scarlet fever cannot be contracted from someone suffering from smallpox. Conversely, another disease can never bring about smallpox. For example, a person suffering from scarlet fever can never cause smallpox in another person. Childbed fever is different. This fever can be caused in healthy patients through other diseases. In the first clinic it was caused by a discharging medullary carcinoma of the uterus, by exhalations from a carious knee, and by cadaverous particles from heterogeneous corpses. In the maternity ward of the St. Rochus Hospital it originated because of decaying matter from the surgical ward, etc. However, childbed fever cannot be transmitted to a healthy maternity patient unless decaying animal-organic matter is conveyed. *[108]* For example, suppose a patient is seriously ill with a form of childbed fever in which no decaying matter is produced. Then the disease cannot be transmitted to healthy patients. On the other hand, if the patient with childbed fever has septic endometritis or discharging metastases, then her disease can be conveyed to healthy patients.

This explains why the conflict over whether childbed fever is or is not contagious could never be conclusively resolved. Those who believe in contagion cite cases in which childbed fever had undeniably spread from an ill patient to a healthy one. Their opponents cite cases in which the disease did not spread as it would have done if it had been contagious. Childbed fever is not a contagious disease, but it can be conveyed from diseased to healthy patients by decaying animal-organic matter. After death, the corpses of puerperae, like all corpses, are sources of the decaying matter that causes the disease.

I assert that in the overwhelming majority of cases childbed fever is caused by external infection and that these cases can be prevented. If we disregard all these cases and also all deaths during maternity that are not due to childbed fever, how many patients are left that die from childbed fever through self-infection? *[109]* As yet, I am not able to provide numbers with which to answer this question. The three institutions in which I made my observations did not adopt those prophylactic measures that are necessary to avoid all cases of external infection. The petition, part of which I quoted earlier, was intended to help me procure a new maternity hospital that would avoid all such cases. Should my petition prove fruitful, and should I have the opportunity over a longer period of years to make observations in such a hospital, it would be possible to determine the number of cases of unavoidable self-infection. Otherwise I must leave it to another more fortunate colleague to determine.

[110] For the present, I accept as a standard the mortality rate of the Viennese maternity hospital from the time before adoption of the anatomical orientation. In the eighteenth century, and in the first decades of the nineteenth century, there were twenty-five years in which not even one patient in one hundred died. [Semmelweis provides a list of twenty-five years between 1786 and 1822 in which the mortality rate ranged from one in one hundred to one in four hundred. After summarizing the list he continues:] *[111]* This small mortality rate may not be the smallest possible. Some of the patients may have died from diseases other than childbed fever. Moreover, even then there could have been infection from external sources; for example, ichor from

diseased patients could have been conveyed to healthy patients. This did in fact occur even before Viennese medicine adopted an anatomical orientation, since even then mortality occasionally reached the rate of 4 percent. The Viennese maternity hospital opened in 1784. Of its first thirty-nine years there were twenty-five during which less than 1 percent died, seven during which 1 percent died, five during which 2 percent died, one year (1814) in which 3 percent and one year (1819) in which 4 percent died. Subject to the above reservations, the twenty-five years within which less than 1 percent died can be adopted as a standard for the frequency of self-infection.

[112] If we judge my results against this standard, it becomes apparent that I was not always successful in restricting the disease to unavoidable cases of self-infection. Occasionally there were cases of external infection. In the last seven months of 1847, in spite of chlorine washings, 56 of 1,841 patients died (3.04 percent). In 1848, when chlorine washings were used throughout the year, 45 of 3,780 patients died (1.19 percent). In January and February of 1849, 21 of 801 patients died (2.62 percent). If we consider individual months, then during only seven months did we successfully restrict deaths to cases of self-infection. Of 276 patients in March 1848 and of 261 patients in August 1848 not a single patient died; in five other months less than 1 percent died. The requirements for the prophylaxis of childbed fever were certainly not met by the construction of the first clinic; this prevented me from limiting deaths to cases of self-infection. *[113]* Moreover, at the time I first arrived at my new convictions, I was myself so inexperienced that in October 1847 I did not wash with chlorine after examining a discharging medullary carcinoma of the uterus, and in November 1847 I did not isolate a patient with a discharging carious knee. [Semmelweis reviews other incidents that caused childbed fever in his practice.]

CHAPTER 3

Etiology

[114] In discussing the concept of childbed fever, I asserted that every case of the disease, without exception, comes about by the resorption of decaying animal-organic matter. I claimed that in the majority of cases this matter is brought to the individual from external sources and that in only a few cases it is produced internally. For me, therefore, the etiological factors of childbed fever include only those which convey decomposing animal-organic matter to the individual from without or which generate this matter internally. Earlier, we examined the accepted etiological factors of childbed fever as an explanation for the increased mortality in the first clinic. We must now determine to what extent these factors can either bring decaying animal-organic matter to the individual or generate it internally. *[115]* We will admit as causes only those factors that do one of these; other factors must be rejected.

Today, the commonest opinion among physicians is that childbed fever consists in a disintegration of the blood and that the anatomical products of childbed fever are excretions from the disintegrated blood. I share this conviction. Epidemic and endemic influences, emotional disturbances, mistakes in diet, and catching a cold have all been claimed to cause the blood to disintegrate. We will now examine these claims. . . .

[116] We begin with epidemic influences. My unshakable conviction is that there are no epidemic influences sufficient to cause childbed fever, that there never have been epidemic causes, and that the endless series of epidemics recorded in medical literature consists entirely of instances of infection from external sources which could have been prevented. The considerations that give me the courage to contradict an opinion so many centuries old

are the following: the ground, the unshakable rock, on which I erect my teaching is the fact that from May 1847 until the present day, 19 April 1859, that is for over twelve years, in three different institutions, I succeeded in limiting childbed fever to isolated cases. Even the most recalcitrant advocates of the epidemic concept are unable to call this an epidemic. And even when the number of deaths increased, it could be proven that the increased mortality was not an epidemic, due to atmospheric-cosmic-terrestrial influences, that is, but rather that it was always due to decaying animal-organic matter transmitted to individuals in spite of my precautions. *[117]* There can be no defense against childbed fever that is due to atmospheric-cosmic-terrestrial influences. Advocates of the epidemic theory secure themselves behind this indefensibility; they thereby escape all responsibility for the devastations of the disease. I myself am impotent against such influences. I do not know what can be done to remove patients from destructive atmospheric-cosmic-terrestrial influences. Thus, if I am successful in preventing a disease long regarded as unpreventable, this proves that the disease is not due to inescapable atmospheric-cosmic-terrestrial influences, and that the cause of the disease is preventable.

The great mortality that is cited by advocates of the epidemic concept does not prove the existence of epidemic influences. . . . *[118]* Suppose that in a specific time many individuals become ill and die of the same disease. As I have indicated, this does not warrant calling it an epidemic. Otherwise, every battle would be an epidemic; in every battle many individuals suffer and die from the same disorder. The concept of an epidemic involves the cause of childbed fever and is completely independent of numbers. Only those cases of childbed fever that are due to atmospheric-cosmic-terrestrial influences are epidemic. . . . It is obvious that epidemic influences bring no decaying animal-organic matter to individuals. However, it is conceivable that atmospheric-cosmic-terrestrial influences result in the production of such matter in many individuals at a given time, that this is then resorbed, and that childbed fever results through self-infection. Such childbed fever would indeed be epidemic. . . . However, if childbed fever were caused by epidemic influences, then, as is observed with other epidemics, it must be limited to a particular season. Opposing atmospheric influences could not have the same results. *[119]* We have proven that childbed fever is not associated with a particular season. Childbed fever occurs in both large and small numbers during each month of the year. . . .

[120–21] The prevailing opinion is that winter is the season most conducive to outbreaks of childbed fever. [Semmelweis refers to earlier tables that prove that] winter really is more frequently an unhealthy time for patients. But this is not to be explained by winter atmospheric influences, since then childbed fever would never occur in larger numbers in summer. It is rather to be explained by the different activities of those who visit the maternity hospital. These activities are determined by the season. After the long vacation in August and September, students resume their studies, including obstetrics, with renewed diligence. In winter the influx of students into the maternity hospital is so great that individuals must wait weeks and even months for their turn to study. In summer, during vacation, half or even two-thirds of the places are vacant. In winter, the pathological and forensic autopsies and the medical and surgical wards in the Imperial Hospital are visited industriously by those who also visit the maternity hospital. In summer, the diligence is noticeably less. The charming surroundings of Vienna are more attractive than the reeking morgue or the sultry wards of the hospital. In winter the assistant of obstetrics holds practical operative exercises on cadavers before the afternoon rounds at four o'clock, because in the mornings students are otherwise engaged, and following the afternoon rounds, at five o'clock, it is already too dark. *[122]* In summer the heat is too oppressive before the afternoon visit, and the operative exercises are held in the evening following afternoon rounds. Does it make any difference to the health of examined patients whether students make rounds before or immediately after they dissect cadavers? These circumstances generally make winter unhealthy and summer healthy for the patients. Suppose we assume that the atmospheric influences of winter really make winter an unhealthy time for patients. Then, assuming that over the twenty-five years when the mortality rate was below 1 percent there were no winter epi-

demics, must one not suspect that through twenty-five years Vienna had no winter? . . .

[123] Just as, if childbed fever were dependent on atmospheric influences, it would be limited to certain seasons, so too the disease would appear only in those climates typified by the weather of that season. In reality it appears in large numbers in all climates. Moreover, in all climates there are maternity hospitals in which it does not appear in large numbers. This appearance and nonappearance of large numbers of cases in different climatic areas cannot be explained by atmospheric influences. It can only be explained by decaying animal-organic matter. In maternity hospitals in different climatic zones where individuals are infected from external sources, childbed fever appears in large numbers and is then falsely called an epidemic. . . .

Irrespective of the climate, favorable health among maternity patients indicates that the hospital is not a teaching institution. The reason for this is obvious. Hospitals that are not teaching institutions but in which individuals are, nevertheless, infected from external sources constitute an exception. . . . *[124]* The Vienna paid maternity ward, a ward for confinement births, belongs in this category. Not only is this ward not used for teaching, but to achieve its purpose it is hermetically closed to all persons other than the physicians employed there. One can, therefore, assume that in this ward there would be no cases of infection from external sources, and as a result, there would be less than 1 percent mortality. However, a glance at the mortality rates for this ward in Table 10 indicates something different. The mortality rate was actually larger than this. A few hours or days after delivery, patients were often released healthy, or occasionally even unhealthy, so that they could return home or be admitted to the general hospital. After I adopted chlorine washings, the health of maternity patients even in the disparaged first clinic was superior to that of patients in the paid ward.

[125] This will cease to be mysterious once I explain these circumstances: the directors of this ward were [Eduard] Mikschik and [Baptist Johann] Chiari.[1] The reader who is familiar

1. Baptist Johann Chiari (1817–54) was Professor of Obstetrics in the Univer-

[124] TABLE 10

	Births	Deaths	Rate
1839	202	6	2.9
1840	204	6	2.9
1841	249	7	2.8
1842	358	10	2.7
1843	367	19	5.2
1844	362	8	2.2
1845	311	6	1.9
1846	315	3	0.9
1847	258	3	1.1
1848	213	4	1.8
Total	2,839	72	
Avg.			2.5

with medical literature will know what these physicians have accomplished. But these accomplishments were possible only through activities in which their hands must have become contaminated with decaying animal-organic matter. Both physicians were simultaneously directors of the gynecological ward of the general hospital. How dangerous a gynecological ward can become for a maternity ward was proven by the discharging medullary carcinoma of the uterus that in October 1847 led to devastation in the first clinic. In the Viennese general hospital between 600 and 800 forensic autopsies are performed each year. The custom is that on alternate weeks one or the other of the two youngest head physicians has to be present as a legal witness. When Mikschik was named chief physician, he was the youngest. After his departure, Chiari was the youngest. Thus, each was obliged to attend the forensic autopsies every other week. Is the unhealthy condition of the maternity patients in the paid ward still mysterious?

Patients in maternity hospitals that are simultaneously teaching institutions are less healthy than those not in teaching institutions. Among teaching institutions, those restricted to educat-

---

sity of Prague and later for a short time in the Josephinum of Vienna. He was the son-in-law of Johann Klein. He supported Semmelweis from the beginning, but also expressed reservations. Semmelweis was generally favorable in his comments about Chiari.

ing midwives have more favorable mortality rates than those restricted to educating physicians. *[126]* This is because the curricula are so arranged that student midwives do not contaminate their hands with decaying matter as often as medical students do.

The Maternité in Paris is an exception. It is exclusively for the education of midwives, but it has a mortality rate as great as [Paul-Antoine] Dubois's Paris Clinic for the education of physicians. Dr. [Franz Hektor] Arneth[2] has said of the location of Dubois's Clinic, "It is regrettable that the autopsy room of the hospital is so near."[3] The Maternité has a mortality rate comparable to that of Dubois's Clinic. [Semmelweis gives tables showing the mortality rates of the two institutions.] *[127–28]* In the Maternité, the curriculum is such that midwives contaminate their hands with decaying matter as frequently as would be the case elsewhere only among physicians. [Johann Friedrich Osiander describes the Maternité as follows:]

> The hospital midwives and some of their students accompanied the physician on his daily rounds through the infirmary for maternity patients. Each student was assigned a diseased patient for particular observation and was expected to prepare a short case history of the birth and of the physician's treatment. . . . *[129]* . . . Autopsies were conducted in a building in the garden somewhat removed from the maternity hospital; these were usually attended by student midwives. I was often astonished to see the active part some of the young women took in the dissection of corpses. With bare and bloody arms, holding large knives in their hands, laughing and quarreling, they cut the pelvis apart, having received permission from the physician to prepare the corpse for him.[4] . . .

2. Franz Hektor Arneth (1818–1907) was assistant in the second clinic while Semmelweis was assistant in the first clinic. Arneth gave favorable lectures on Semmelweis in Paris and in London. After spending some time in Russia, Arneth became a successful practitioner in Vienna.

3. Franz Hektor Arneth, *Über Geburtshülfe und Gynäkologie in Frankreich, Grossbritannien und Irland* (Vienna [Braumüller], 1853), [p. 51; author's note].

4. Johann Friedrich Osiander, *Bemerkungen über die französische Geburtshülfe, nebst einer ausführlichen Beschreibung der Maternité in Paris* (Hannover: Hahn, 1813), pp. 33, 46 [author's note].

[130] . . . The reader can understand how the midwives in the Maternité contaminate their hands with decaying matter.[5]

If childbed fever were due to atmospheric-cosmic-terrestrial influences, then it would be impossible for there to be a so-called epidemic of childbed fever in some hospitals and for other hospitals in the same climatic zone to be spared. Over a long period of time, it would be even more unlikely for these influences to devastate, in varying degrees, the two divisions of one hospital. *[131]* Table 1 shows that through six years the maternity patients in the first clinic in Vienna died at a rate consistently three times greater than the patients in the second clinic. This observation first made me doubt the epidemic concept of childbed fever.

The same inequality of mortality between two divisions of one institution occurred in Strasbourg. Dr. Arneth writes that in Strasbourg,

> The maternity hospital consists of two divisions, the clinic for physicians and the division where midwives are trained. Until the end of 1845 the two divisions were under different directors; they were next to one another, separated only by a thin wall. Admissions were arranged so that maternity patients went alternately into the two divisions. During the vacation all were accepted into the clinic. Since [Charles Henri] Ehrmann left, both divisions have been directed by [Joseph-Alexis] Stoltz. It is not possible to determine the precise mortality rates, but both professors agree that the clinic for male students has consistently more deaths.[6]

For more precise information I wrote to Dr. [Friedrich] Wieger[7] and Professor Stoltz in Strasbourg, and received the following replies. Dr. Wieger wrote:

5. It was always possible for midwives to become contaminated with decaying matter. In a lecture in 1846 Kolletschka is reputed to have said, "It is here no uncommon thing for midwives, especially in the commencement of their practice, to pull off legs and arms of infants, and even to pull away the entire body and leave the head in the uterus. Such occurrences are not altogether uncommon; they often happen." *Lancet* 2(1855): 503.

6. Arneth, op. cit., note 3 above, p. 30.

7. Wieger had been Semmelweis's student in the first clinic and was, in his own words, an eyewitness to Semmelweis's discovery; he also wrote a positive report on Semmelweis's work that appeared in a French medical periodical. Judging

[132] . . . What Arneth has told you is correct. During the time that the midwife school was under Professor Ehrmann, puerperal fever was relatively unknown. At that time both divisions were housed in wings in the third floor of the large hospital, separated only by a room containing the beds of students who lived in the building. When Professor Stoltz took over both divisions, the disease became common in both, and it remains so. The divisions are now united in an attractive, newly erected pavilion.[8]

Professor Stoltz writes:

. . . The passage in Arneth's book . . . is accurate, but I have always attributed the difference in mortality to the sanitation of the two divisions. In fact, the rooms of the faculty clinic are inferior, less spacious, and always overcrowded, while the midwives' rooms are well-ventilated, well-appointed, and contain proportionately fewer beds. They are also kept cleaner, and in the course of a year they contain fewer pregnant and diseased patients. *[133]* The more difficult cases are always assigned to the faculty clinic.

Until 1856 both divisions were part of the general hospital. Last year they were moved into a single, well-situated building facing south and west, and surrounded by courtyards and a garden. The two clinics are separated by a lecture hall and a room for instruments. Pregnant women are given places on the ground floor. The division for midwives is still more conveniently arranged than that for the faculty. Nevertheless, in the winter of 1856–57, here as in Munich, there was an equally fatal and devastating epidemic in both divisions. This is in spite of the fact that the faculty clinic employed chlorine for disinfecting hands.

You see, honored colleague, that our observations of your theory of the etiology of puerperal fever have not been favorable. I will, nevertheless, read with great interest your work on these matters and attempt to follow painstakingly all your prescriptions.

I am delighted to have entered into this scientific correspondence with you, and I will be pleased if it is not limited to this one occasion.[9] . . .

---

by Stoltz's comments below, however, Wieger either failed to grasp the significance of Semmelweis's work or he did not have a significant influence on his associates.

8. Strasbourg, 19 May 1858 [author's note].

9. Strasbourg, 26 March 1858 [author's note].

[134] . . . Does it not contradict good sense to insist that childbed fever, which before the unification of the two divisions was limited to the division for physicians, is epidemic, that is, dependent on atmospheric-cosmic-terrestrial influences? Professor Stoltz himself sought the cause of childbed fever in endemic noxious influences, particularly in the difference in sanitary conditions between the divisions. However, the more favorable conditions of the division for midwives did not protect it from childbed fever, because those conditions were nullified once it ceased to be exclusively for midwives. Also, in the new building, the more favorable conditions of the division for midwives did not protect it from childbed fever. . . . *[135]* Judgment about the ineffectiveness of the chlorine washing will be reserved for another part of this work.[10]

Before the Strasbourg school for midwives was unified with the division for physicians, and from the time the Viennese second clinic was devoted exclusively to midwives until adoption of chlorine washing in May 1847, these two proved that patients are healthier in teaching institutions where only midwives are trained than in institutions for training physicians.

The great mortality rate in maternity hospitals is not dependent on atmospheric conditions but rather on decaying animal-organic matter. This must be true, since so-called epidemic childbed fever began in various hospitals when decaying matter was first conveyed to patients in a specific, regular way. Osiander relates that the Maternité in Paris was horribly ravaged by childbed fever in 1803 and in 1808. We find in the educational system of the Maternité a sufficient etiology. Between 1803 and 1808 in Vienna less than 1 percent died from childbed fever; there the so-called epidemic of childbed fever began in 1823. This was the time when Viennese medicine adopted an anatomical orientation. *[136]* Professor Rokitansky has functioned at the Institute for Pathological Anatomy since 1828. For twenty-four years, from 1823 until chlorine washings began in 1847, mortality al-

10. In discussing the reaction to his work, Semmelweis later points out that opponents to his theories are not likely to use chlorine conscientiously and that their unfavorable results, therefore, are not a reliable indication of the usefulness of his methods. See below, pp. 194f.; German edition, pp. 330–32.

ways exceeded 2 percent and was sometimes as high as 12 percent. During the thirty-nine years from 1784 through 1822 mortality never exceeded 4 percent, and in twenty-five years it was less than 1 percent. In a letter that I will later quote in full, the late [Gustav Adolf] Michaelis wrote from the Kiel maternity hospital, "Puerperal fever first appeared here in 1834. That is, however, approximately the time when I first became active in instruction and when students began examining regularly." Epidemic childbed fever first appeared in the Strasbourg school for midwives in 1845, the year in which it was united with the division for physicians. In the St. Rochus Hospital in Pest the health of maternity patients has been continuously unfavorable since the existence of the obstetrical division. This is because the maternity ward was an appendage to the surgical division. However, the health of the maternity patients of the medical faculty of Pest was always good until the 1840s. In Pest, medicine adopted an anatomical orientation at that time.

My predecessor, Councilor [Ede Flórián] Birly,[11] once Boër's assistant, believed that his maternity patients in Pest were healthier than those in Vienna because of his extensive use of purges. He believed that childbed fever was caused by uncleanliness of the bowel. At the opening of his clinic each October he regularly directed a stinging oration against Vienna and claimed that the great mortality rate in Vienna was due to their negligence in the administration of purgatives. *[137]* However, as soon as medicine in Pest became anatomically oriented, the purgatives lost their prophylactic powers. At a time when I was not yet a member, the College of Medical Professors in Pest was repeatedly obliged to close the clinic during the school year because childbed fever became so overwhelming. I cannot provide figures, because the records were lost in the [1848] revolution. I live in the city about which I speak, and this is sufficient guarantee that I speak the truth.

The great mortality in the maternity hospitals is not depen-

11. Ede Flórián Birly (1787–1854) preceded Semmelweis as Professor of Theoretical and Practical Obstetrics at the University of Pest. He never accepted Semmelweis's opinions although he and Semmelweis worked together closely for four years.

dent on atmospheric influences, but rather on decaying matter that is regularly transmitted to patients from external sources. This follows from the fact that when circumstances are changed so that decaying matter is less frequently transmitted, mortality declines. . . . If the spread of decaying matter is completely halted, epidemic childbed fever is also halted. An example is the maternity ward in St. Rochus Hospital in Pest. It was separated from the surgical division and placed under my direction. *[138]* For six years I had no epidemic, even without chlorine washing. . . . If measures are adopted to destroy decaying matter, the so-called epidemics of childbed fever cease, even though they may have been raging for years. Examples are the first clinic in Vienna and the obstetrical clinic in Pest. Foreign experience supporting this will be discussed later.[12] . . .

[139] The mortality for the two clinics in the eight years from 1833 until 1841, during which male and female students were divided equally between both clinics, is shown in Table 11. I regret that I am late in obtaining the facts reported in this table and that I could not include this information where I first needed it. The reader may want to reread [pages 94 and 95 above; German edition,] pages 63 and 64.[13] . . .

In the years following adoption of the chlorine washings, the mortality rates in the two clinics are as given in Table 12.

[140] Even I have not achieved the smallest possible mortality rate. This will be discussed in the appropriate place below.[14] Evaluation of the increased mortality [in the years after I left the clinic] will be delayed until we discuss the failure of chlorine washings as attempted by other obstetricians.[15] *[141]* It is sufficient here to note that all the physicians officially functioning at this time in both clinics were and are opposed to my opinion regarding the origin of childbed fever. My successor, Carl Braun, wrote against my opinion. Carl Braun's successor, his brother

12. In discussing reaction to his work Semmelweis mentions several foreign cases in which adoption of chlorine washing reduced mortality. See below, pp. 174f., 186, 188–90; German edition, pp. 283–88, 307, 310–13.

13. See above, chap. 1, footnote 17.

14. See below, pp. 163f.; German edition, pp. 266f.

15. See below, pp. 193–95; German edition, pp. 330–32.

[139] TABLE 11

	First Clinic			Second Clinic		
	Births	Deaths	Rate	Births	Deaths	Rate
1833	3,737	197	5.29	353	8	2.26
1834	2,657	205	7.71	1,744	150	8.60
1835	2,573	143	5.55	1,682	84	4.99
1836	2,677	200	7.47	1,670	131	7.84
1837	2,765	251	9.09	1,784	124	6.99
1838	2,987	91	3.04	1,779	88	4.94
1839	2,781	151	5.04	2,010	91	4.05
1840	2,889	267	9.05	2,073	55	2.06
Total	23,066	1,505		13,095	731	
Avg.			6.56			5.58

[140] TABLE 12

	First Clinic			Second Clinic		
	Births	Deaths	Rate	Births	Deaths	Rate
1847	3,490	176	5.00	3,306	32	0.09
1848	3,556	45	1.27	3,319	43	1.33
1849	3,858	103	2.06	3,371	87	2.05
1850	3,745	74	1.09	3,261	54	1.06
1851	4,194	75	1.07	3,395	121	3.05
1852	4,471	181	4.00	3,360	192	5.07
1853	4,221	94	2.02	3,480	67	1.09
1854	4,393	400	9.10	3,396	210	6.18
1855	3,659	198	5.41	2,938	174	5.92
1856	3,925	156	3.97	3,070	125	4.07
1857	4,220	124	2.92	3,795	83	2.18
1858	4,203	86	2.04	4,179	60	1.43
Total	47,935	1,712		40,770	1,248	
Avg.			3.57			3.06

Gustav, has disclosed his opinions by 400 deaths in 1854. In the seventy-five years of the maternity hospital even the combined deaths of both clinics exceeded this figure only three times—in 1842 with 730 deaths, in 1843 with 457 deaths, and in 1846 with 567 deaths. . . .

To provide a clear overview of the health of the patients cared

[142] TABLE 13

	Before Separation of Clinics		
	Births	Deaths	Rate
Before pathological anatomy	71,395	897	1.25
After pathological anatomy	28,429	1,509	5.30

	After Separation of Clinics					
	First Clinic			Second Clinic		
	Births	Deaths	Rate	Births	Deaths	Rate
Male and female students Equally divided between clinics	23,059	1,505	6.56	13,097	731	5.58
Students divided by sex, before chlorine washings	20,042	1,989	9.92	17,791	691	3.38
After chlorine washings	47,938	1,712	3.57	40,770	1,248	3.06
Total	91,043	5,206		71,656	2,670	
Avg.			5.71			3.72

	Births	Deaths	Rate
Total for all seventy-five years	262,523	10,282	
Avg. for all seventy-five years			3.91

for in the Viennese maternity hospital, in Table 13 I show the most important figures for the crucial time periods.

[142–45] Table 13 must persuade every disinterested person that deaths in the Viennese maternity hospital were dependent on decaying animal-organic matter. This table shows clearly that variations in mortality were determined by the frequency with which decaying matter was conveyed from external sources. Since the laws of nature are the same throughout the entire world, I conclude that atmospheric-cosmic-terrestrial influences are never capable of inducing childbed fever. The endless series of epidemics reported in medical literature consists of cases of preventable infection from without; in other words, all these cases of the disease originate through the introduction of decaying animal-organic matter.

So-called epidemics in the maternity hospitals are not due to atmospheric influences but rather to decaying animal-organic matter. This is proven by the healthier condition of patients in countries where English opinions dominate, as in Ireland and Scotland. There is no basis for assuming that the atmospheric influences that supposedly destroy patients in German and French hospitals do not also exist in England, Scotland, and Ireland. *[146]* Thus atmospheric influences cannot explain the difference in health of the patients in these lands. However, English physicians are significantly different from the French and Germans in their opinions regarding the origin of childbed fever. The English regard childbed fever as contagious; in France and Germany, childbed fever is not believed to be contagious. I do not believe that childbed fever is contagious; however, healthy patients can be infected by decaying matter that is generated in diseased patients. Childbed fever is not conveyed from all diseased maternity patients, only from those who generate decaying matter. After death, childbed fever can be conveyed from every corpse to a healthy patient providing that the corpse has decayed sufficiently.

The English, proceeding from the opinion that childbed fever is contagious, will not visit a healthy maternity patient if they have earlier visited one who is ill unless they first wash with chlorine and change their clothing. If the number of diseased patients increases, they travel or give up their practice for a time. After an autopsy of a puerperal corpse, English physicians will not visit healthy maternity patients without first washing in chlorine and changing their clothing. *[147]* In those cases where ill patients do not generate decaying matter, English physicians take superfluous steps. But after treating ill patients who do generate such matter, English physicians, seeking to destroy a contagium, destroy that which, if conveyed to healthy patients, would cause childbed fever. . . .

In a significant essay Chiari claimed that in many cases decaying matter can be drawn from these sources.

[148] I call attention to a condition that, although frequently discussed, nevertheless requires more explanation. This is the origin and prevention of so-called puerperal epidemics. I say so-called because it has been established that this disease does not occur in many cases simultaneously over a large district, but usually only in institutions for delivery, and also not equally in different divisions of the same institution. I will not return to the different opinions regarding the causal origin of this really horrible disease. However, I will offer a few observations regarding the cause of many cases of the disease among maternity patients. These observations were made in connection with my responsibilities in Prague.

Because of an unusually thick cervix, a first delivery was protracted from 23 through 27 January 1853. Gangrene ensued. After useless baths, douches, antiphlogistic measures, and incisions in the swollen, cartilaginous and finger thick cervix, the dead fetus was cut in order to reduce its size and to end the four-day birth process. During the last two days, secretions from the vagina were brownish and very bad smelling. The patient became seriously ill with septic endometritis and died on 1 February. While this patient was in the delivery room, nine other patients became ill; all but one died. They had all been in the delivery room at the same time. *[149]* From the end of January many cases of illness followed until, from May through October, the health of the patients improved.

I became convinced that in this concrete case the cause of the frequent illnesses was the spread of gangrenous matter from the diseased patient to healthy ones. Naturally, all possible caution was observed in order to avoid spreading harmful matter through examinations. Nevertheless, the simultaneous residence of one ill patient and of several healthy ones in the same relatively small locality makes it possible for harmful matter to be spread in various ways. Given that several persons became ill, it is conceivable that in an institution where space is inadequate for numerous births the disease may be propagated in this way. I do not wish to imply that all so-called puerperal epidemics must arise in this way. However, I wish to call attention to a condition that may and will frequently occur in large institutions for delivery.

In confirmation of my opinion I had a second tragic experience. In October 1853, a few days before my return to Prague after a vacation, it became necessary to perform surgery on a woman who had been in labor for several days because of a narrow pelvis. This patient died of septic endometritis with inflamed synchondrosis [certain cartilaginous joints, in this case probably those located in the pubic region (symphysis pubica)]. From then on several serious cases of disease were encountered; they ceased only in the middle of November. From then until the end of my stay in Prague, namely until the end of August of the next year, I was fortunate enough not to observe more cases of this horrible disease.

[150] By these observations I intend to show only that by careful attention one is sometimes able to establish the mode of origin of numerous cases of disease in maternity hospitals. Moreover, this method of origin was already identified by Semmelweis. Also this autumn, in the clinic for midwives, a similar observation was made and privately communicated to me by my friend Dr. [Joseph] Späth.[16]

I regard it a matter of conscience to publish these observations. For even though I have not said that this is the only way in which this plague can originate, nevertheless, these retrospective observations can have great practical significance in the organization of maternity institutions. It is imperative that in larger maternity institutions several delivery rooms be held ready in order that cases of protracted delivery can be isolated from ordinary deliveries. It is self-evident that this isolation is necessary also in the organization of instruction. In consequence of my opinion that the spread of maternity diseases in large institutions depends on transferrence of foul harmful matter, I sought opportunities to avoid this cause. I employed the following preventive measures: first, I divided instruction so that individual patients were never examined by more than five students, after which every participant was required to wash his hands with chloride of lime. *[151]*

16. Joseph Späth (1823–96) was Professor of Obstetrics in Vienna and from 1873 until 1886 he was director of the Second Obstetrical Clinic. Semmelweis regarded him as a principal opponent. By 1864, however, he had adopted Semmelweis's view, and observed that virtually all obstetricians were convinced that Semmelweis was correct, although few admitted it openly. Frank P. Murphy, "Ignaz Philipp Semmelweis (1818–65): An Annotated Bibliography," *Bulletin of the History of Medicine* 20(1946), 653–707: 669f.

Second, so that students could not easily come to the clinic from anatomical work, I conducted the clinic both summer and winter in the morning hours between seven and nine. Third, I watched very closely that the laundry was cleaned conscientiously. Because of the second epidemic, vulvar compresses were washed outside the hospital. Fourth, it was easily comprehendible, for example, that by sponging the ulcerated genitals of a patient, this condition could be transmitted to other patients. Thus I adopted the policy of cleansing the genitals of patients only by sprays rather than by sponges. Although sponges do come into contact with the genitals, it is much less likely that sprays will. Fifth, I sought to remove the seriously ill from the maternity wards by transferring them into the general hospital. This measure was also necessary because space was limited. Everyone must see that it is very much to the purpose, from both physical and moral considerations, to prevent the accumulation of such diseased patients in the maternity institution. Sixth, from the opinions expressed above, it also followed that when many people became diseased in a maternity institution, it became necessary to change location. Even the furnishings of a hospital could provide the means by which disease was spread.

It therefore appeared advisable that new institutions should be so constructed that, for example, each obstetrical clinic would be located in its own building and, even in respect to the laundry, completely isolated from other clinics. *[152]* Since as a result of utilizing these measures insofar as possible frequent cases of puerperal disease ceased after one or two months, I believe myself able to recommend them most enthusiastically.[17]

From Chiari's observations the reader sees that many cases of disease can be caused by the decaying matter generated by one diseased patient. Decaying matter generated by patients is not the only source of so-called puerperal epidemics, however. This follows from what I have said about the sources of this matter.

Patients are healthier in maternity hospitals where it is believed that childbed fever is contagious and where steps are taken to destroy the contagion. This follows from a report published by Professor [Karl Edouard Marius] Levy of Copenhagen. The

17. [Baptist Johann] Chiari, "Winke zur Vorbeugung der Puerperal-Epidemie," *Wochenblatt der Zeitschrift der k. k. Gesellschaft der Ärzte zu Wien* [11] (1855): [117–21; author's note. Semmelweis quotes the entire article.]

report concerns the maternity hospitals and the teaching of practical obstetrics in London and Dublin. Professor Michaelis in
Kiel has translated the report. I cannot resist reproducing the
introductory remarks of the translator.

> [153] On a recent trip I had the opportunity to convince myself
> of the truth of the present report. The industriousness and thor-
> oughness of the report must also convince every reader.
>
> The author's main object is to explore the conditions under
> which puerperal fever appears and the techniques that have been
> successfully used to control it. English institutions offer the most
> important results in this matter, for whereas they were formerly
> devastated by this plague, mortality in London and Dublin insti-
> tutions has been reduced to just over 1 percent through the adop-
> tion of health measures in the last decades. Unfortunately, on the
> continent we are still a long way from such favorable results. . . .
> With the advance of education and of human sensitivity [*Human-
> ität*] public opinion is being forcefully aroused—even in places
> where formerly there was indifference to this horrible offering of
> human life. The goal is clear: one must make the institutions
> healthy, or close them. . . .
>
> [154] For those with experience in the matter, no proof is re-
> quired for the assertion that this plague will not be extinguished
> through therapeutic treatment. Thorough and strictly observed
> measures of cleanliness, ventilation, etc. offer more hope. Indeed,
> according to the experience of the British, this approach will cer-
> tainly lead to success. . . .
>
> Fortunately, in Vienna last year it was discovered that the dis-
> ease could be reduced significantly by cleaning the hands with
> chlorine before examining. With time, use of this remedy re-
> duced the number of deaths to nearly one-tenth the normal rate;
> an obviously striking result. We owe this discovery to Dr. Sem-
> melweis, who will certainly soon publish the details. Apparently,
> the use of this remedy, together with universal disinfection, will
> usher in more fortunate times for our maternity hospitals. [155]
> I must publicly thank Dr. [Heinrich] Hermann Schwartz of Hol-
> stein for bringing the Viennese experience to my attention.—Kiel,
> 17 April 1848.[18] . . .

18. The original essay by Karl Edouard Marius Levy appeared in *Bibliothek
for Laeger*, the German translation [entitled "Gebärhäuser und der praktischen
Unterricht in der Geburtshülfe"] by [Gustav Adolf] Michaelis was published in
Neue Zeitschrift für Geburtskunde 27 [(1850):, 392–449; author's note].

[Next come six pages of tables showing that three British maternity hospitals had mortality rates usually ranging between .5 and 2 percent. Semmelweis observes that a midwife, Mrs. Widgen, attributed a higher mortality rate of 4.93 percent in one hospital to an autopsy that was performed in the hospital that year. Next, there is a table of annual mortality rates for another British hospital—in this case mortality averaged over 3 percent over several years, and then, through 1844, 1845, and 1846, it was reduced to zero. Semmelweis quotes Levy's discussion of this change.]

[156–61] . . . In the immediate neighborhood of the building, not 30 feet from the wall, an open pit was found that was more than 1,500 feet in area. This pit received the refuge from the adjacent poor and densely built part of the city. The contents of the pit were stagnant, and boiled constantly through the production of gas. In 1838 after numerous difficulties and debates with the water commission, the hospital administration finally succeeded in having a 644-foot stretch of the pit cleaned and covered. In the process, however, one mistake occurred—instead of carrying away an incredible hulk of black, stinking slime, it was simply spread nearby on the ground. This, of course, greatly increased the surface of evaporation. Within twenty-four hours two cases of puerperal fever occurred in the hospital; Dr. [Edward] Rigby believed that they could be traced directly to this irresponsible procedure. . . . *[162]* [In 1838, while all this was going on, the hospital had a mortality rate of 26.76 percent. Then, while the mortality rate remained high, a new ventilation system was installed. The mortality rate declined significantly, and some of the physicians were inclined to attribute the decline to this new system. However, Levy notes, doubts remained because] now and then a stinking mass of liquid had been observed to surface in the cellar near the hearth of the smokestack. Investigation disclosed that the water was coming from the drainage system. The building's drains were examined. The main drain was found to be so firmly blocked by some pieces of wood that it seemed to have been done intentionally. The whole surrounding area of the cellar was abundantly strewn and saturated with filth and it was impossible to determine how long this condition had existed.[19]

[Semmelweis quotes more of Levy's discussion of whether the

19. Ibid., pp. 418–20.

decline in mortality was due to a change in the ventilation system or to the correction of the unsanitary conditions. Semmelweis remarks that given either possibility, the disease was not due to atmospheric-cosmic-terrestrial influences. Semmelweis reproduces several more of Levy's tables showing favorable mortality rates for British, Irish, and Scottish hospitals. Semmelweis then observes] *[163–68]* . . . We have examined eight maternity hospitals throughout three countries. In seven of these, mortality just exceeded 1 percent; in the eighth it was 3 percent. We do not find the causal moment for this larger mortality in atmospheric influences but rather in the harmful matter of the drainage canals that surrounded the building.

Why should atmospheric influences so strikingly spare maternity hospitals in the United Kingdom while so many patients in German and French hospitals are sacrificed? The answer is that there are no atmospheric influences to which German and French patients are falling victim; rather decaying animal-organic matter is being brought to the individuals from external sources. This causes the mortality in the hospitals of the United Kingdom and of France and Germany. Because of the circumstances of the French and German hospitals, decaying matter is much more frequently transmitted to patients in those hospitals, and they have a greater mortality rate. *[169]* In the United Kingdom, individuals are much less often exposed to decaying matter from without, thus their mortality rates are much lower. The English regard childbed fever as contagious. Thus they employ chlorine washings and destroy the decaying matter taken from ill patients and from corpses. In German and French maternity hospitals this matter is not destroyed. As Chiari has shown, this can cause many cases of illness. In German and French hospitals decaying matter is frequently taken from corpses and from ill persons who are unaffected by childbed fever. As a rule German and French maternity hospitals are associated with large general hospitals. Therefore their students occupy themselves in morgues, and in medical and surgical wards, as well as in maternity wards. In this way they become carriers of the decaying matter that initiates so much misfortune. Maternity hospitals in the United Kingdom are independent institutions; because they are removed from general hospitals, the students are forced to concern themselves exclusively with obstetrics.

Some may attribute the favorable health of the London maternity hospital to the fact that there are never more than two students training at one time. But I must observe that students do not constitute atmospheric influences and that childbed fever caused by students with contaminated hands is not, therefore, epidemic childbed fever. *[170]* It clearly matters whether many or just a few students with contaminated hands examine patients, but it does not matter whether many or a few students with clean hands examine patients. This is proven by the Dublin maternity hospital; Levy writes: ". . . A practical school has been established where, in the course of time, several thousand young physicians from all parts of England have sought a practical education in obstetrics. This finally proves that it is only cowardly superstition to discount the needs of education and science and to assert that a horrible death rate is the unavoidable result of large maternity institutions." [20] This is also proven by the first clinic in Vienna where, in April 1847, without chlorine washing and with only twenty students, 57 of 312 patients died (18.27 percent), while in 1848, with chlorine washings and with forty-two students, 45 of 3,556 died (1.27 percent). In order to clarify the difference in mortality rates between maternity hospitals in which individuals contaminate themselves with decaying matter at different rates, in Table 14 we will compare the reports of the Dublin and Viennese maternity hospitals for a period of sixty-six years. Both are institutions for the education of physicians.

[172–78] . . . The great mortality in the maternity hospitals is not dependent on atmospheric influences, since delivering women among the general population do not simultaneously suffer from childbed fever. The maternity hospital and the surrounding area must be subject to the same atmospheric influences. *[179]* However, while patients in the hospital are decimated, other women enjoy good health. This is proven by the measure of closing the maternity hospitals; after a hospital is closed, births do not cease,

20. Ibid., p. 449

but women give birth in various locations rather than being admitted to a hospital. Those who deliver remain healthy; in nearby maternity hospitals they would be killed by atmospheric influences. Certainly many women giving birth die outside maternity hospitals. But these deaths cannot be attributed to atmospheric influences. This is true, since increased mortality outside the hospitals is not always simultaneous with that in the hospitals. The mortality in the hospitals is often high while it is low outside, and high mortality outside the hospitals is very rarely observed.

Childbed fever outside the maternity hospitals—exactly like that which rages inside—is, without exception, a resorption fever dependent on the resorption of decaying animal-organic matter. In exceptional cases, both inside and outside the maternity hospitals, the decaying matter is created within the attacked individual and childbed fever originates through self-infection. In the overwhelming majority of cases, however, the decaying matter is transmitted to the individual from external sources; childbed fever then originates as external infection, whether in or out of the hospitals. *[180]* Both inside and outside maternity hospitals, physicians who practice obstetrics perform autopsies and treat patients who are generating decaying matter. . . . Midwives cleanse patients who are producing decaying matter. . . . *[181]* . . . However, private physicians have fewer opportunities to contaminate their hands, so childbed fever is less common outside maternity hospitals. . . . The busy physician may only care for a few obstetrical cases each day. In the Viennese maternity hospital, there are often thirty or forty births within twenty-four hours. Therefore, a private physician whose hands are contaminated cannot cause as many cases of childbed fever as can a physician in a large maternity hospital. Moreover, outside the hospital, individuals are generally examined by only one physician; in the hospital, a person may be examined by many. Although one unclean hand is sufficient to cause many deaths, with many examining hands it is more likely that one hand or another will be contaminated.

Arneth has published a very informative collection of experi-

	Dublin Maternity Hospital			Viennese Maternity Hospital		
	Births	Deaths	Rate	Births	Deaths	Ra
				BEFORE SEPARATION OI CLINICS Before Pathological Anatomy		
1784	1,261	11	0.87	284	6	2.
1785	1,292	8	0.61	899	13	1.
1786	1,351	8	0.59	1,151	5	0.
1787	1,347	10	0.74	1,407	5	0.:
1788	1,469	23	1.56	1,425	5	0.:
1789	1,435	25	1.74	1,246	7	0.!
1790	1,546	12	0.77	1,326	10	0.˙
1791	1,602	25	1.56	1,395	8	0.!
1792	1,631	10	0.61	1,579	14	0.!
1793	1,747	19	1.08	1,684	44	2.(
1794	1,543	20	1.29	1,768	7	0.:
1795	1,503	7	0.46	1,798	38	2.˙
1796	1,621	10	0.61	1,904	22	1.˙
1797	1,712	13	0.75	2,012	5	0.:
1798	1,604	8	0.49	2,046	5	0.:
1799	1,537	10	0.65	2,067	20	0.˙
1800	1,837	18	0.97	2,070	41	1.˙
1801	1,725	30	1.74	2,106	17	0.:
1802	1,985	26	1.30	2,346	9	0.:
1803	2,028	44	2.16	2,215	16	0.˙
1804	1,915	16	0.83	2,022	8	0.:
1805	2,220	12	0.54	2,112	9	0.
1806	2,406	23	0.95	1,875	13	0.˙
1807	2,511	12	0.47	925	6	0.(
1808	2,665	13	0.48	855	7	0.:
1809	2,889	21	0.72	912	13	1.˙
1810	2,854	29	1.01	744	6	0.:
1811	2,561	24	0.98	1,050	20	1.˙
1812	2,676	43	1.69	1,419	9	0.(
1813	2,484	62	2.49	1,945	21	1.(
1814	2,508	25	0.99	2,062	66	3.:
1815	3,075	17	0.51	2,591	19	0.˙
1816	3,314	18	0.54	2,410	12	0.
1817	3,473	32	0.92	2,735	25	0.˙
1818	3,539	56	1.58	2,568	56	2.
1819	3,197	94	2.94	3,089	154	4.˙
1820	2,458	70	2.84	2,998	75	2.
1821	2,849	22	0.77	3,294	55	1.
1822	2,675	12	0.44	3,066	26	0.

	Dublin Maternity Hospital			Viennese Maternity Hospital		
	Births	Deaths	Rate	Births	Deaths	Rate
				After Pathological Anatomy		
1823	2,584	59	2.28	2,872	214	7.45
1824	2,446	20	0.81	2,911	144	4.98
1825	2,740	26	0.64	2,594	229	8.82
1826	2,440	81	3.33	2,359	192	8.12
1827	2,550	33	1.29	2,367	51	2.15
1828	2,856	43	1.50	2,833	101	3.56
1829	2,141	34	1.59	3,012	140	4.64
1830	2,288	12	0.52	2,797	111	3.97
1831	2,176	12	0.55	3,353	222	6.62
1832	2,242	12	0.58	3,331	105	3.15
				AFTER SEPARATION OF CLINICS Males and Females in Both		
1833	2,138	12	0.56	3,737	197	5.29
1834	2,024	34	1.67	2,657	205	7.71
1835	1,902	34	1.78	2,573	143	5.55
1836	1,810	36	1.98	2,677	200	7.47
1837	1,833	24	1.30	2,765	251	9.09
1838	2,126	45	2.11	2,987	91	3.04
1839	1,951	25	1.23	2,781	151	5.04
1840	1,521	26	1.70	2,889	267	9.05
				Males in First Clinic Only		
1841	2,003	23	1.14	3,036	237	7.07
1842	2,171	21	0.96	3,287	518	15.08
1843	2,210	22	0.99	3,060	274	8.09
1844	2,288	14	0.61	3,157	260	8.02
1845	1,411	35	2.48	3,492	241	6.08
1846	2,025	17	0.83	4,010	459	11.04
				Chlorine Washings Used in Physicians' Clinic		
1847	1,703	47	2.75	3,490	176	5.00
1848	1,816	35	1.92	3,556	45	1.27
1849	2,063	38	1.84	3,858	103	2.06
Total	141,903	1,758		153,841	6,224	
Avg.			1.21			4.04

ences of the English regarding the origin of childbed fever outside the hospital.

> *[182]* Puerperal fever is such a frightful disease that we must be
> interested in what English physicians think of the disease in gen-
> eral, and especially how they treat patients, and what they think
> about its most mysterious aspect—its etiology.
>
> During a non-epidemic period, the experienced [John] Rober-
> ton classified women according to the frequency with which they
> were attacked by puerperal fever. According to his experience,
> those who care for a household are visited by the disease much
> less frequently than those who are served. In the industrial city
> of Hulme, only a small number of the 40,000 inhabitants retain
> servants. The far greater number of the female inhabitants are
> working women who arise at five in the morning, send the older
> children to work, and either accompany their husbands to the
> factories or are busy from early in the morning until late at night
> conducting the household and caring for children. Throughout
> pregnancy, even as the first phrase of delivery approaches and is
> endured, such women must continue the same activities until se-
> rious labor pains force them to stop. In spite of such depriva-
> tions, official records for the decade 1839–49 indicate that only 1
> of 196.5 deaths was due to childbed fever. In four small neigh-
> boring villages whose inhabitants were much more leisured, 1 of
> 84 deaths was due to this cause. *[183]* Of course the situation is
> quite different during an epidemic; crowded together in small
> rooms with numerous other local inhabitants, poor maternity pa-
> tients frequently die. The prosperous, living in greater comfort
> and cleanliness and with conscientious care, enjoy much greater
> hope. In Roberton's opinion the unhealthy aspects of both social
> classes apparently unite in the wives of shopkeepers and small
> merchants. These pass their days in poorly constructed houses
> and in spite of their better training, coddling, and amusements
> are not able to enjoy the advantages of the more prosperous classes.
>
> We will investigate numerous experiences in England which
> suggest that puerperal fever can be induced in delivering women
> by the transmission of gangrenous foul matter in general, and of
> particles from corpses in particular. However, as we will see, these
> cases have usually been interpreted quite differently. Among the
> various articles and editorials that have appeared in England, none
> showed more insight than a journal article by Robert Storrs. Storrs

asked various colleagues for their experiences and opinions. The results of his queries included the following: [G.] Reedal in Sheffield treated a young man who suffered and finally died from an open tumor and an erysipelatous infection.[21] *[184]* . . . While Reedal cared for the patient, five women whose deliveries he attended between 26 October and 3 November 1843 contracted puerperal fever and died. He visited these unfortunate women almost immediately after attending to the wounds of the former patient. Two other women, at whose deliveries he also assisted, did not become ill, but he did not visit them until a few hours after the dangerous call. After these deaths Reedal ceased visiting the young man, because he recognized that he himself was the carrier of the disease. Since then he has had no more cases of puerperal fever than he had before treating the case of erysipelas. Mr. [R. P.] Sleight of Hull records that while treating a patient for erysipelas, he was called to attend a delivery. The delivery proceeded normally; nevertheless, within twenty hours the woman succumbed to puerperal fever, and she died eighteen hours later. [Semmelweis, still quoting Arneth, relates several more similar stories.]

[185–87] . . . Storrs hopes to have proved: *[188]* (i) that puerperal fever is communicable through physical contact, (ii) that puerperal fever derives from an animal poison and, in particular, from erysipelas and its sequelae, and occasionally from typhoid, (iii) that without differences in the circumstances of the patient, childbed fever brings about erysipelas, typhoid, and in men a fever that sometimes is remarkably similar to puerperal fever, and (iv) that the most rapid, conscientious, and informed treatment remains without success. Storrs recommends that to avoid mishaps, obstetricians should never visit persons in labor while wearing the same clothing formerly worn when attending other patients. This concerns especially the outer clothing that usually carries the matter which generates the disease. Once erysipelas or typhoid is encountered, the same measures must be adopted for all maternity patients. After autopsy or an operation on a person suffering from erysipelas or typhoid, the surgeon must always

---

21. Erysipelas is a contagious disease of the skin and subcutaneous tissues now known to be an infection by a particular streptococcus. It was particularly common following surgery and often accompanied the other symptoms of puerperal fever. The British regarded it as related to puerperal fever and, therefore, as particularly dangerous to puerperae.

wash as carefully as possible and change his clothing completely before attending a delivery. One must not disregard gloves because the hands and arms are the parts of the body most likely to convey the poison. *[189]* Once the disease is established in a physician's practice, he should leave his residence for two or three weeks, change his entire wardrobe, wash everything conscientiously, and avoid every case of illness that could serve as a source of the animal poison.

A similar communication from Roberton generated a great sensation in England. A midwife who had a considerable practice among beneficiaries of a particular charitable society had the misfortune to be present when a woman she delivered died of puerperal fever. In the following month, December 1830, she attended deliveries of 30 women from different parts of the city, and 16 died of childbed fever. This circumstance was particularly striking because 380 other deliveries were performed successfully at the same time by other midwives from the same organization. The physicians of the institution persuaded the midwife to discontinue her practice for a time and to go into the country. Within a short time puerperal fever was encountered in the practices of other midwives and physicians at various points throughout the city. By June the disease raged with a distribution and fury that had never been known in Manchester. . . .

[190–91] . . . In contrast to Semmelweis and Skoda, the English do not conclude that putrid matter has been conveyed to the sexual organs of the women. They conclude that the disease *qua talis* is conveyed from one woman to another. Thus [Fleetwood] Churchill remarks, "After carefully examining the facts, I cannot doubt that the disease spreads through infection and contact, i.e., that from one person suffering from puerperal fever it can be conveyed to another whom the first touches or has as a neighbor."

Deciding which interpretation is correct may be of great practical importance. Given the opinion common in England, one need not proscribe contacting corpses of persons who die from diseases other than puerperal fever. On the other hand, given the assumption that a healthy person cannot convey the disease without having touched an ill one, one can feeely go from an ill maternity patient to others without changing clothing as is required in England. The English assume that it is possible to convey the disease for a fairly long time; thus they frequently recommend that a physician who encounters numerous cases of puerperal fever should temporarily give up assisting at births and should change his entire wardrobe. *[192]* This is justified by citing occurrences where numerous cases of puerperal fever arise in the practice of one physician or midwife while other physicians have no similar cases. This circumstance can be explained more easily if one assumes that these physicians have been involved either with autopsies or with other putrescent substances, the opening of abscesses, cleaning and binding of wounds, cleaning or examining maternity patients, extracting placentas, etc. Many physicians have temporarily interrupted their obstetrical practices after losing several women to puerperal fever. Upon resuming their practice after a period of several weeks they were not more fortunate; this proves that the cause they identify is not responsible.[22]

[193] I am also convinced that the activities of physicians cause puerperal fever. I include this information to demonstrate that activities outside the maternity hospital can also cause childbed fever. However, I draw conclusions different from those drawn by English physicians.

I regard childbed fever as a non-contagious disease because it cannot be conveyed from every patient with childbed fever to a healthy person, and because a healthy person can contract the disease from persons not suffering from childbed fever. Every victim of smallpox is capable of giving smallpox to healthy people. A healthy person can contract smallpox only from one who has smallpox; no one has ever contracted smallpox from a person suffering from cancer of the uterus. This is not the case with childbed fever. If childbed fever takes a form in which no decaying matter is produced, then it cannot be communicated to a healthy person. However, given a form that produces decaying matter, as for example septic endometritis, the disease is certainly communicable. . . . Moreover, childbed fever may come from diseased states other than childbed fever, for example from gangrenous erysipelas, carcinoma of the uterus, etc. *[194]* . . . A contagious disease is conveyed by the matter which is produced only by that particular disease. . . . Puerperal fever is

22. Arneth, [op. cit., note 3 above], pp. 334–44 [author's note].

conveyed by matter that is the product not only of childbed fever but also of the most heterogeneous diseases. Every corpse,
no matter what the cause of death, produces matter that can cause
childbed fever. It follows that one must avoid contacting corpses
or diseased patients who produce decaying matter, whether or
not they are puerperae. A veterinarian who is simultaneously an
obstetrician could draw from diseased or dead animals decaying
matter that would cause childbed fever in maternity patients.

Thus childbed fever is not a contagious disease, but it is a
disease that can be conveyed to a healthy person by means of
decaying matter. Childbed fever bears the same relation to erysipelas and its sequelae that it does to every other disease that
generates decaying matter. Childbed fever stands in the same
relation to erysipelas and its sequelae that it does to every decomposing corpse. In recognizing only erysipelas and its sequelae, beyond puerperal fever itself, as sources of childbed fever,
English physicians draw the boundaries much too narrowly. This
is shown by the cases previously discussed.

[195] Thus childbed fever is the same disease that occurs among
surgeons and anatomists, and following surgical operations, it is
the same disease whether decaying matter is brought into the
circulation system of males or of females. The decaying matter
is not resorbed through the epidermis or through a thick layer
of epithelium; in surgeons and anatomists resorption must be
preceded by a wound. As a qualified pathological anatomist,
Kolletschka had his hands contaminated with decaying matter
on countless occasions and he nevertheless remained healthy.
Through a prick, resorption was made possible; we know which
disease was the consequence. The site of resorption can be any
point on the body that is stripped of epidermis and epithelium.
The inner uterine surface of maternity patients has neither epidermis nor epithelium; this is the site of resorption of the decaying matter that causes childbed fever. If injuries occur during
birth, any part of the genitals, indeed any wounded part of the
whole body, can be the site of resorption. In the school year
1857–58 at the obstetrical clinic in Pest, the outer genitals of two
maternity patients became gangrenous. One of the students assigned to care for these patients had a small abrasion on one

finger from a needle prick. She contracted lymphangitis with suppuration of the auxiliary glands and was seriously ill for several months.

[196] For patients in the maternity hospitals the genital region is generally the only area suitable for resorption; thus, in order to contract childbed fever, it is necessary that decaying matter be transmitted to the genital area. Since the clothing of the obstetrician does not contact the genitals, the English custom of changing clothes is a harmless but superfluous measure. In 1848 in Vienna, the students and I did not change clothing after activities with objects suitable to induce childbed fever. We only exposed our hands to the operation of chlorine, and in 1848 of 3,556 patients we lost only 45 (1.27 percent) to childbed fever. In cases cited above, an obstetrician visited healthy patients without having changed clothing and his patients died of childbed fever. It was not the clothing but the hands that carried decaying matter. Since hands cannot be changed, they must be disinfected. If clothing became contaminated with decaying matter, the hands were certainly still more contaminated, and it is with the hands that one makes internal examinations.

In order for childbed fever to occur, it is a *conditio sine qua non* that decaying matter is introduced into the genitals. With the exception of internal obstetrical examinations, an individual can carry out every possible medical examination with contaminated hands without the slightest danger. The epidermis prevents the resorption of decaying matter. Obstetricians carry the matter on their hands for hours and even days without harming themselves. [197] If this matter is brought into contact with the inner surface of the uterus, even for a moment, it is resorbed and childbed fever results. The hands of the anatomist are often in contact with decaying corpses for hours at a time and he remains healthy. If the epidermis is removed by an injury, however, the disease is generated—this happened to Kolletschka and to the student midwife.

Because of the arrangement of the rooms in the first clinic, general rounds were made twice daily in the following order: first was the visit to the labor room, where half the healthy patients were examined; then the diseased patients were examined;

and finally the remaining half of the healthy patients were visited. Suppose in visiting the diseased patients we contaminated our hands. If, without having washed in chlorine, we had then taken the pulses of healthy patients, if we had felt their abdomens externally, in a word, if we had made all the necessary medical examinations with the exception of internal obstetrical examinations, we would not have propagated childbed fever. Childbed fever cannot be induced through external unwounded surfaces of the body. Therefore, it is not spread as is smallpox when the outer surface of a healthy individual comes within breathing distance of a diseased person. Of course, if the exhalations of a diseased individual enter the uterus, then the disease is certainly spread.

[198] We noted that changing clothing after visiting a diseased patient is harmless but superfluous. Clothing can cause childbed fever only when its exhalations enter the uterus with the air, and clothing is not easily contaminated to this degree. Clothing could also cause childbed fever if, for example, the cuff of one's jacket is contaminated with decaying matter and contacts the genitals during the birth. This, however, is not a common happening. In this sense clothing certainly can be harmful, but not in the way the English believe. They hold that puerperal contagium, like smallpox contagium, can be conveyed on clothing to a healthy patient and that it is then absorbed through the outer surfaces of the body, thereby causing childbed fever. . . . [199] . . . I have clearly indicated how my opinion concerning the nature and spread of childbed fever differs from the opinion of English physicians. . . .

It was once a mystery how an epidemic disease could also be brought about through trauma. Knowing now that puerperal fever comes about through resorption of decaying matter, this is no longer a mystery. After a difficult operation with forceps, certain parts of the genitals may be crushed and become necrotic. If these necrotic parts are resorbed, childbed fever is caused by self-infection.

The geographical distribution of childbed fever proves that it is not caused by atmospheric influences but rather by contact with external decaying matter. [Conrad Theodor Carl] Litzmann writes,

[200] Most epidemics known to us are limited to central Europe. Notes about epidemics outside Europe are incomplete; they include observations on childbed fever from [Hugh Lennox] Hodge in Philadelphia and from Scholz in Jerusalem. Generally cold and moist lands appear especially afflicted; for example, England is more seriously afflicted than France. The same holds for cities on the banks of large rivers, for example, Vienna. On the other hand, according to Brydone's report, women in Sicily seldom become ill after delivery. Savary reports in his letters from Egypt that nursing diseases are entirely unknown there, and Dr. Salles reports that during his three-year visit to South America he saw no cases of childbed fever. Nevertheless, these reports are too incomplete to warrant conclusions. Probably childbed fever is spread over the entire world, and its frequency depends less on climate than on the presence or absence of large cities, in particular of large maternity institutions.[23]

Being convinced that childbed fever originates by the resorption of decaying matter, I interpret Litzmann's remarks as follows. Certainly in isolated cases of self-infection, childbed fever occurs throughout the world. Also, throughout the world there are diseased persons whose diseases generate decaying matter and who are treated by the same medical personnel who assist deliveries. Consequently, childbed fever occurs occasionally throughout the world because of infection. *[201]* Certainly childbed fever would be more frequent if individuals were more frequently infected with decaying organic matter. However, this happens only in central Europe where there is occasion for handling decaying matter and where there is opportunity for many persons in maternity hospitals to be infected. Childbed fever is particularly associated with large cities because large maternity hospitals are found there. The cities do not cause childbed fever, since childbed fever can be suppressed by closing the hospitals and by allowing women to be delivered in the cities themselves.

The puerperal epidemic in Vienna was not caused by Vienna's location on the banks of a large river, since for twenty-five years less than 1 percent of Viennese patients died of the disease. Moreover, the use of chlorine washings did not make the Dan-

---

23. C. T. Carl Litzmann, *Das Kindbettfieber in nosologischer, geschichlicher und therapeutischer Beziehung* (Halle: [Eduard Anton], 1844), p. 129 [author's note].

ube dry, but the epidemic ceased. If the Danube had caused the epidemic in Vienna, why would the epidemic appear in Vienna but not in all the other places along its banks? If childbed fever does not occur in Sicily, Egypt, and South America, it is certainly not because they lack water. Rather it is because in these areas pathological anatomy, the pride of the Viennese school and the scourge of the Viennese maternity hospital, is not yet dominant.

[202] Published reports of the English maternity hospitals indicate an average mortality of 1 percent; the French lose 4 percent. Thus Litzmann is simply wrong in claiming that England is more subject to childbed fever than France.

The history of childbed fever proves that it is not caused by atmospheric influences but rather by the spread of decaying matter. In his history of childbed fever, in which all the epidemics before 1841 are reported, Litzmann writes:

> Insofar as existing historical documents permit one to judge, childbed fever is a modern disease. The cases reported by Hippocrates that are generally identified as such do not belong to this classification. There are only examples of bilious fever, then common, which among maternity patients was no different from its appearance among non-maternity patients or men; Hippocrates himself never identified it as a separate and distinguishable disease. Pain in the right hypochondrium, bilious diarrhea and vomiting, headache with delirium or fainting, fever with more or less frequent irregular chilling constitute the symptoms common to all these cases. It is not noted, as a basis for differentiation, that among maternity patients there is a disruption in puerperal secretions. In only three cases do we find a suppression of lochia, and in two of these, pain in the area of the uterus is mentioned. In recent times [Theodor] Helm has shown that recurring chilling, from which several of the ill suffered, in connection with the disease in question, indicates metrophlebitis [inflammation of the veins of the uterus].

> *[203]* . . . We encounter the first, as yet unclear indication of childbed fever in the second half of the seventeenth century at the Hôtel-Dieu in Paris. [Phillipe] Peu relates that mortality among the newly delivered was very great and greater in certain seasons than others. The year 1664 was particularly devastating. This

striking mortality was attributed to the fact that the maternity rooms were directly over the hall where the wounded were situated. The mortality of the maternity patients was in direct proportion to the number of wounded. In humid weather, warm or cold, the rate was higher; in dry weather it was variable. By changing the location of the maternity patients to the lower floor the disease was eliminated. The description is highly deficient and tells only that the patients were subject to hemorrhages and that their corpses were full of abscesses.[24]

Osiander gives us more precise disclosures regarding the Hôtel-Dieu and the prevalence of childbed fever there.

In the noteworthy report of the hospitals of Paris which [Jacobus-Rene] Tenon prepared for the government in 1788, we read that the lower abdominal infection, *la fièvre puerpérale*, had raged every winter since 1774 among the maternity patients of the Hôtel-Dieu, and that often as many as 7 of every 12 patients suffered from it. *[204]* This is less surprising if one knows the deficient conditions then endured by patients in the Hôtel-Dieu. They were enclosed in the upper story in low-ceilinged, small halls overcrowded with beds. Three patients would often lie next to one another in a bed four feet wide. In 1786, 175 pregnant and newly delivered women and 16 attendants slept in sixty-seven beds of ordinary width. Moreover, the hall for maternity patients was directly over other sick rooms. Thus while the wounded were not, as formerly, directly under the maternity patients, one can certainly assume that the proximity of large halls for the diseased contributed to the corruption of the air and to the creation of a dangerous miasma in the halls for maternity patients.[25]

Thus, the first recognized epidemic of childbed fever was not caused by atmospheric influences but rather in the way that I have taught. Perhaps no historians can be found to reveal the mystery of the countless remaining puerperal epidemics. In any case, historians do record autopsy results from each respective epidemic; this reveals the source from which the epidemic drew its existence. *[205]* I have described how epidemics began at the

24. Ibid., pp. 130f.
25. Osiander, [op. cit., note 4 above,] p. 243 [author's note].

Viennese maternity hospital, at the maternity ward at St. Rochus, and at the obstetrical clinic at Pest. By using these descriptions as a guide, perhaps one can dispel the mystery surrounding other epidemics in maternity hospitals.

The history of epidemics at the Viennese maternity hospital proves that the frequency and virulence of epidemics are directly related to the development of the anatomical orientation in medicine. In 1789 Boër entered his teaching post and, in 1822, was succeeded by Professor Klein. Boër, the reformer of obstetrics, the author of [a textbook on] natural obstetrics, was discouraged because of what was then regarded as an enormous mortality rate, and he retired prematurely from his post. Yet in twenty-one years Boër lost less than 1 percent of his patients, in six years he lost 1 percent, in four years 2 percent, in one year 3 percent, and in one year 4 percent. How horribly has the anatomical orientation increased the mortality rate! Between 1822 and 1858, even including the years when chlorine washing was employed, the mortality rate was the following: one year 0 percent, three years 1 percent, six years 2 percent, four years 3 percent, six years 4 percent, four years 5 percent, three years 6 percent, four years 7 percent, five years 8 percent, and one year 12 percent. . . .

[206]. . .It is unimportant whether the cases cited by Hippocrates were childbed fever. Only a few cases were involved, and these could have occurred by self-infection. Alternatively, they may have been cases of infection from external sources; certainly even in Hippocrates' time there were sick people whose diseases generated decaying matter, and there were also male and female medical personnel who treated these diseased persons along with women who were pregnant and in labor. In this way external infection was possible. Boër says this of Hippocrates:

> One is filled with reverence and astonishment, when treating puerperal fever and opening corpses of those who died from it, when contemplating the course and consequences of the disease, which Hippocrates reported so truly and appropriately more than 2,000 years ago. If every century could produce one physician so observant, rather than so many who are educated in theoretical systems, how much more would have been achieved for human-

ity and for animal life generally. *[207] The Book of Women's Diseases* contains from paragraph sixty nearly to paragraph ninety an historical description of all those forms under which puerperal fever sporadically manifests itself. *The Book of Epidemics* contains observations regarding its epidemic manifestations that are so accurately and masterfully depicted that it could not have been done more correctly had it been recorded yesterday at bedside or in the dissection room.[26]

From the success of the chlorine washings I am convinced that atmospheric influences have not brought about the endless series of puerperal epidemics. The cases reported in the medical literature are all avoidable cases of infection from without. Readings in the history of childbed fever confirm this perfectly.

I will now recapitulate the facts that have convinced me that there are no atmospheric-cosmic-terrestrial influences capable of causing childbed fever, and that there never have been such influences. . . . The most important reason is that in three different institutions I greatly reduced mortality by destroying decaying matter. This could not have been done if atmospheric influences caused childbed fever. *[208]* The disease appears in large numbers in every season; this is not compatible with the atmospheric concept of childbed fever, but the reason is clear as soon as one knows that childbed fever arises from external infection. . . . Atmospheric influences cannot explain why hospitals are spared for many years while later, for many more years, they are afflicted annually with so-called epidemics of childbed fever. . . . *[209]* Atmospheric influences cannot explain why different divisions in one and the same institution have different conditions of health, or how it happens that maternity patients in the city at large are healthy while patients in hospitals suffer from epidemic childbed fever, or why to save these patients it is necessary to close the maternity hospitals and to force these women to be delivered in the city. Atmospheric influences cannot explain why, at a given time, different maternity hospitals in the same city have different conditions of health. But all this is

26. [Rogers] Lucas Johann Boër, *Abhandlungen und Versuche zur Begrundung einer neuen, einfachen und naturgemässen Geburtshülfe* (Vienna: [von Mösk], 1810), [vol. 2, pp. 3f.; author's note].

clear once we know that childbed fever originates by the spread of decaying matter. . . .

At the first clinic during a six-year period the mortality rate was three times as great as in the second clinic, although the clinics were separated only by a common anteroom. In Strasbourg two wards were separated only by a room containing the beds of student midwives, but the wards had significantly different mortality rates. *[210]* In the Maternité childbed fever raged as early as the end of the eighteenth century; in Vienna it began in 1823. In Dublin during ninety-eight years mortality reached 3 percent in only two years. In seven maternity hospitals in England, Ireland, and Scotland the mortality rate averaged only 1 percent. According to the epidemic theory of childbed fever, atmospheric influences which cause the disease are spread over whole continents. . . . How can such a theory be brought into harmony with the observed distribution of the disease? Why were atmospheric influences that already afflicted the Maternité at the end of the eighteenth century so slow in being extended to Vienna? How did these influences finally come to operate more furiously in Vienna than in Paris? How is it that these influences were so weakened in England, Scotland, and Ireland? Given that the Viennese clinics shared a common anteroom, what barrier protected the second clinic so successfully from influences that were otherwise spread over the whole continent? . . . *[211]* . . . As soon as one knows that childbed fever arises from decaying matter which is conveyed from external sources, explanations are easy. . . .

Out of respect for obstetricians I prefer to believe that until now no one has attempted to reconcile the epidemic theory with these universally known facts. I cannot believe that anyone seriously interested in the truth can continue to believe in the epidemic theory after its disharmony with these facts becomes apparent. *[212]* Anyone who has been confronted by these facts and who, nevertheless, continues to believe in epidemic childbed fever does not have the courage to acknowledge the truth. Perhaps such persons fear that upon recognizing the truth a great guilt is imputed. However, the facts cannot be changed, and denying the truth only increases guilt. Those who continue to believe in epidemic childbed fever can have no conviction or comprehension, they carry in their minds only memorized words.

The doctrine of epidemic childbed fever explains the unknown with the unknown. There are many deaths; we know not why. One seeks to explain these by unknown atmospheric influences, but one cannot specify any particular influences, since childbed fever occurs in every season and in every climate.

These are the reasons for my conviction. For the sake of humanity, I wish that everyone who reads this may derive the same conviction. To spare further review, those considerations that are advanced in support of atmospheric influences and that have not yet been refuted will be examined in the course of criticizing my opponents.

CHAPTER 4

Endemic Causes of Childbed Fever

[213] Overcrowding in maternity hospitals is an endemic cause of childbed fever only because in a crowded hospital it is more difficult to maintain the necessary degree of cleanliness and to isolate dangerous individuals. Overcrowding can foster the creation and spread of decaying matter in these ways. However, when the necessary degree of cleanliness is observed, so that no decaying matter is created, or when dangerous individuals can be isolated, or when no dangerous persons happen to be present, it does not matter whether a maternity hospital is crowded. [Semmelweis provides forty-four pages of tables to prove that the mortality rate in the Viennese hospital was not related to the degree of overcrowding. This largely repeats Table 3 above.]

[214–58] We have not yet considered puerperal miasma, because in the first clinic this was never used to explain the mortality rate. [For the sake of completeness] we will now do so. If several healthy patients and their infants are in one room, the air becomes saturated with skin odors, milk secretion, lochial discharge, etc. If these exhalations are not promptly removed through ventilation, they begin to decompose. If the decomposed exhalations penetrate the genitals of the patients, childbed fever can result. If diseased patients are in a room and if decaying matter is exuded by them, it can become mixed with the air in the room and penetrate the genitals of the patients and can cause childbed fever. *[259]* If this is what one understands by puerperal miasma, then I do not object; anything else that may be understood by puerperal miasma is non-existent. To protect against the decomposition of physiological exhalations it is sufficient to ventilate by opening windows. To protect healthy patients from the ex-

halations of decaying matter from diseased patients, the diseased patients must be isolated.

Since the creation of puerperal miasma supposedly depends on the number of patients present, the preceding tables showing that mortality is not dependent on overcrowding also prove there is no creation of puerperal miasma. This also follows from the fact that I significantly reduced mortality in the first clinic without taking any precautions to destroy puerperal miasma. The only prophylaxis for childbed fever was washing the hands with chlorine.

Puerperal fever does not generate a contagium, it produces a miasma only in the sense previously mentioned, and it cannot be contracted through uninjured outer body surfaces. It follows that puerperal fever does not infect a hospital so that healthy patients become infected merely by being there. *[260]* There can be few places where more maternity patients have died than in the sick room of the first clinic. After I initiated chlorine washings, the sick room was only occasionally required, so it was used as a maternity room. But without tearing out the floor or scraping down the walls, and after only changing the beds, the patients cared for in this room remained healthy. A location can bring forth childbed fever only if it becomes so polluted with decaying matter that the exhalations of the decaying matter saturate the air and penetrate the genitals of the individuals therein. A dissection room could become contaminated to this degree, but rooms in a maternity hospital could not.

Fear is not a causal factor in childbed fever; fear can neither transmit decaying matter to an individual nor cause it to be generated internally. As I mentioned, fear cannot explain the origin of the high mortality rate in the first clinic, because fear comes only as a consequence of such a mortality rate. Similarly, I was totally unable to prevent patients from being afraid, but nevertheless they became healthier. They were admitted with the same fear but childbed fever declined. If fear were an etiological factor in childbed fever, childbed fever would appear outside the hospitals as frequently as inside; fear is not limited to those who deliver inside the hospital. As every active obstetrician knows, women fear throughout pregnancy that they will not survive delivery; even after many pregnancies they fear that this time they will pay for delivery with their lives. *[261]* In nearly all texts on obstetrics, one reads that particularly toward the end of pregnancy the fear of death embitters the lives of pregnant women. Many fear death ten or twelve times in this way without contracting puerperal fever.

Most of those who deliver in maternity hospitals are single women from the comfortless classes. Throughout pregnancy they have earned their bread by hard work, they have experienced need and suffering, they have been deprived of emotional support, and they have led generally unhappy and dissolute lives.[1] But these circumstances do not infect them with decaying matter, nor do they foster the internal generation of decaying matter. Therefore these factors do not cause childbed fever. Certainly not everyone who delivers in a maternity hospital lives in this way. [Moreover,] if these factors caused the disease, the mortality rate outside the hospital would be larger—not all those who deliver outside the hospitals are happy, virtuous women who spend their days in pleasant living.

It has been proposed that women are embarrassed to deliver in the presence of men and that offended modesty is a causal factor in childbed fever. But offended modesty does not convey decaying matter from without and it does not create it internally. The thoughtlessness of discussions of the etiology of childbed fever is evident here: victims are depicted as dissipated and yet assumed to possess such tender modesty as never appears in the higher classes. *[262]* Women in the highest circles also give birth in the presence of physicians; their offended modesty does not

1. Most of those who delivered in maternity hospitals were unmarried. Physicians often regarded this as of etiological significance. One British physician noted, "In hospitals seduced women are always an easy sacrifice; but, even among the affluent, powerful secret causes of mental depression may act with as much force, and expose them to its influence. Such causes are generally unknown to the physician." Edward William Murphy, "On Puerperal Fever," *Dublin Quarterly Journal of Medical Science* 24(1857), 1–30: 19. These views certainly were related to the idea that puerperal fever was sometimes due to providence. Oliver Wendell Holmes, "The Contagiousness of Puerperal Fever," in *Medical Essays* (New York: Houghton, Mifflin, and Co., 1883), pp. 103, 125.

cause them to die of childbed fever. Because of our system for educating midwives, they are sufficiently trained to assist with most births. Fortunately for both mother and child, only rare cases require the help of an obstetrician. In many lands obstetricians are called only in these rare cases. However, the help that only the obstetrician can provide must often be provided quickly if it is to be of any use. If the obstetrician is not called until danger arises, he often arrives too late to help. Because of such experiences, an obstetrician should attend every birth. If offended modesty were a causal factor in childbed fever, in order to protect a few persons from this sort of danger, every patient would need to be exposed to the threat of childbed fever. If offended modesty were the etiological factor in childbed fever, male obstetricians would have to be forbidden.

Conception, pregnancy, hyperinosis, hydremia, plethora, individuality, dietary mistakes, and chilling are not etiological factors in childbed fever because these factors neither convey decaying matter from without nor foster its generation internally. *[263]* If these were etiological factors, childbed fever would not be limited to central Europe or to modern times.

Conveyers of decaying matter include chief physicians and assistants who, either for their own instruction or in teaching their students, contaminate their hands; the head of a surgical ward who simultaneously directs an obstetrical ward; directors of united gynecological and obstetrical wards; students of practical obstetrics who attend pathological or forensic autopsies or autopsies of persons who die in maternity wards, or who visit surgical wards; students of obstetrics who enroll in courses involving operations on corpses, or who attend courses in the microscopic study of organic tissues; functioning assistants who assign students to perform obstetrical operations on cadavers; assistants and students who perform autopsies; directors of maternity clinics and their assistants who treat diseases in which decaying matter is generated; sick patients who are delivered or treated in rooms in which healthy patients are also delivered or treated; hospital personnel who administer douches to the ill and then examine large numbers of healthy people; the many items, for example sponges, instruments, washing bowls, etc., that are used both for the ill and for the healthy; linen and bed equipment that is not always kept sufficiently clean; air in maternity hospitals that is saturated with decaying matter, either because the exhalations of the patients are not removed by ventilation, or because decaying matter is conveyed to the hospital as, for example, from a nearby morgue or from an open sewage canal. Outside the hospital, the same etiological factors induce childbed fever; for example, medical personnel, male or female, who examine with contaminated hands, or who use contaminated equipment. *[264]* All these are causal factors; many more could be added if it were not superfluous to do so. Everything that brings decaying matter to the individual from external sources belongs in this category. These are the etiological factors that devastate maternity patients—devastations falsely attributed to atmospheric influences.

Etiological factors that can cause an individual to generate decaying matter internally include retention and decomposition of normal lochial discharge; retention of the placenta, or of the remnants of the placenta or its membrane; retention of blood clots in the uterus; and crushing of the genitals during prolonged labor, or in consequence of operations that produce necrosing lacerations in the pelvic tissues. *[265]* Only extended observation can reveal whether there are additional causes of self-infection. Until now my observations have been made in institutions where it was not possible to prevent all infection from without. However, cases of self-infection may be few, since in Vienna of 2,012 patients in 1797 and 2,046 patients in 1798 only 5 patients died each year; 1 in 400.

CHAPTER 5

Prophylaxis of Childbed Fever

[266] The only cause of childbed fever is decaying animal-organic matter that is either introduced to the individual from external sources or generated internally. Thus, the prophylaxis of childbed fever involves preventing the introduction of external decaying matter, preventing the internal generation of decaying matter, and removing as quickly as possible any existing decaying matter or preventing its resorption.

Decaying matter is usually spread in manual examinations. Given a large number of students, it is safer to avoid contamination than to clean what has once been contaminated. I therefore appeal to all governments to proclaim laws forbidding those engaged in maternity hospitals from activities likely to contaminate their hands. The imperative necessity of such laws is made clear by my experience in the first clinic; in spite of all my exertions, I did not succeed in limiting childbed fever to cases of self-infection. [267] Bear in mind that the semester for practical obstetrics does not begin on a fixed day when all can simultaneously be made aware of their responsibilities. Rather, a few students join and leave each day. Because one cannot repeat the same things every day, it can easily happen that many are first warned after they have been there several days. Consider that the forty-two students in the first clinic spend the largest part of their day in the morgue performing pathological and forensic autopsies, in the divisions of the general hospital, in various operations, and in other courses. In all these activities, their hands become not only contaminated but actually saturated with decaying matter. Moreover, although it is difficult to believe, these students will not take the time necessary for chlorine washings to disinfect their hands completely. When one considers these circumstances, it is understandable that there were still cases of infection from external sources in the first clinic.

This evil situation can only be corrected by the law mentioned above. This law would have other beneficial consequences. I will later cite numerous professors of obstetrics who have written against my teaching. Only a fool could believe that students who have been taught so fallaciously will disinfect themselves as conscientiously as necessary. And when death reaps a rich harvest, the failure of chlorine washing is cited as evidence for the epidemic origin of childbed fever.

This pernicious behavior—whereby many human lives are prematurely destroyed, whereby additional generations of misled physicians are sent out into practice, and whereby cases of infection outside the maternity hospitals are then used as evidence that childbed fever is epidemic—can only be ended by such laws. *[268]* If, in consequence of the law, students in maternity hospitals have clean hands, then the most ardent lecture on epidemic influences will no longer cause epidemics. Without this law, such lectures make students careless, and childbed fever is increased by hands contaminated with decaying matter. I therefore implore all governments to proclaim such laws in order that the childbearing sex will not be further decimated, in order that life yet unborn will not be infected with seeds of death by those very persons who are called to protect life. Such a law would not hinder other aspects of medical education, because practical obstetrics is a relatively short course. Moreover, the law would significantly promote the teaching of practical obstetrics, because the most informative cases would no longer occur while students are occupied in other activities. Theoretical obstetrics is used everywhere to introduce instruction in practical obstetrics. Operations on corpses should be part of this theoretical instruction. Students attending lectures on theoretical obstetrics should attend autopsies of those who die in the maternity hospitals. Then, before being admitted into the maternity hospital, they would be familiar with the pathological anatomy of childbed fever and with obstetrical operations on corpses. This would make such activities [as autopsies] unnecessary while students are involved in the hospitals. Such laws would eliminate the most prolific, but by no means the only, activities in which hands become contaminated. Even in maternity hospitals childbed fever can originate through self-infection; when this takes the form of septic endometritis, the hands of the examiner can become contaminated. Also, patients are admitted who suffer from diseases that produce decaying matter. *[269]* Thus it will always be necessary to disinfect the hands.

In order to disinfect the hands completely it is necessary to oil them before they are contaminated so that the decaying matter cannot penetrate the pores. Thereafter the hands must be washed with soap and then exposed to the operation of a chemical agent to destroy the decaying matter. I employ chloride of lime and wash as long as is necessary to make the hands slippery. Hands treated in this way are completely disinfected. Decaying matter is carried not only by the examining finger but also by everything contaminated that can come into contact with the genitals. These items must, therefore, either be disinfected or no longer used.

Because air can also carry decaying matter, maternity hospitals must be built in areas where no decaying matter can be conveyed to them. Thus, maternity hospitals should not be part of large general hospitals. So that air in the maternity hospitals will not carry decaying matter, exhalations of the individuals in hospitals must be removed by ventilation before decomposition begins. It is also necessary that every maternity hospital contain several isolation rooms in order that individuals who exude decaying matter can be isolated. *[270]* It is unimportant how many healthy patients are cared for in one room so long as the number of patients is appropriate for the size of the room. In the first clinic we cared for thirty-two patients in one room.

The prophylaxis of childbed fever does not require that several small maternity hospitals be erected in place of one large one. Certainly total mortality cannot be as great in a small hospital as in a large one; for example, in the maternity clinic at Würzburg, [Franz] Kiwisch [von Rotterau][1] reported 27 deaths

1. Franz Kiwisch von Rotterau (1814–52) was Professor of Obstetrics at the University of Würzburg and later at the University of Prague. He was another of Semmelweis's principal opponents.

from 102 patients cared for during one year. The least favorable year of the seventy-five years of the Viennese maternity hospital was 1842; taking the hospital as a whole, of 6,024 patients 730 died; in the first clinic alone, of 3,287 patients 518 died. What a horrible difference between the total number of deaths in the small hospital in Würzburg and the large one in Vienna. Nevertheless, the relative mortality in the small Würzburg hospital was significantly larger than even the worst year in the largest maternity hospital in the world: in Würzburg 26.47 percent died, in Vienna for the hospital as a whole only 12.11 percent, and in the first clinic alone only 15.75 percent died. It is easy to explain why the relative mortality in smaller maternity hospitals is greater than in large ones. *[271]* In small hospitals the teaching material is restricted and every patient must be used. If they are examined with contaminated hands, a high percentage of the patients will become infected. In Vienna there is such an excess of teaching material that hundreds of individuals are not used for teaching and thus are not infected.

To prevent self-infection, one must prevent decaying matter from being generated internally during delivery. When delivery is prolonged so that the genitals become crushed, it is necessary that the required operation be concluded as quickly as possible. The operation itself must be carried out carefully; otherwise it could result in that very state [death] for the prevention of which the operation was carried out. Thus rotation and pendular movements with forceps, for example, are reprehensible because the genitals are necessarily crushed in the process.

Remnants of the placenta and membrane must be extracted from the organism before they begin to decompose. Several hours after the uterus ceases to bleed, injections must be given in order to remove any clotted blood that remains within; otherwise this begins to decompose and leads to self-infection. One must avoid perineal lacerations, because these provide both a resorbant surface and resorbable matter. Once decaying matter is created it must be removed through cleanliness and injections so that resorption is avoided where possible. To the extent that these circumstances also arise outside the maternity hospital, the same prophylaxis must be observed.

In order that these measures will be observed everywhere, medical personnel must be made to swear in the oath and in the official instructions given when they receive their diplomas that they will conscientiously discharge all that is required by these prophylactic measures. *[272]* Instead of losing 1 patient for every 3 or 4 that are admitted, those who observe these measures may lose as few as 1 in 400—certainly less than 1 in 100.

CHAPTER 6

Reactions to My Teachings:
Correspondence and Published Opinions

[273] If my goal were only to provide an unshakable foundation for my teachings and to make clear the tragic mistakes of the epidemic theory of childbed fever, I would conclude at this point. I have nothing to add to these teachings that will establish them more firmly; neither can the indefensibility of the epidemic theory of childbed fever be made more clear. These are not the sole purposes of this essay, however, for my teaching is not intended to be firmly established while moldering under the dust of the library. Its mission is to achieve benefits in practical life. My doctrines exist in order to be promulgated by teachers of medicine, in order that all medical personnel, even to the last village practitioner or midwife, will behave accordingly. My doctrines exist to rid maternity hospitals of their horror, to preserve the wife for her husband and the mother for her child.

The anniversary of the beginning of my teaching falls in the second half of May; if twelve years after May of 1847 I ask myself whether my teachings have fulfilled their mission, the answer is disappointing. It is true that my teachings have never been presented so fully as on this occasion, but the substance of the theory has been made public; namely, it is a known fact that injuries during autopsies can cause pyemia, and that the findings in the corpses of those who die of pyemia are identical with those in the corpses of persons who die of childbed fever. Thus childbed fever is the same disease. If it is the same disease, it must have the same cause. This same cause is doubtless most frequently to be found on the hands of physicians. If removing the cause prevents the effect, there remains no doubt in the case.

[274] This much was public from the beginning. One would have assumed that for scientists, whose purpose is saving lives, such indications would have been sufficient to warrant serious reflection, especially concerning a disease that everyone agrees is so horrible. One would believe that the clarity of things would have made the truth apparent to everyone and that they would have behaved accordingly. Experience teaches otherwise. Most medical lecture halls continue to resound with lectures on epidemic childbed fever and with discourses against my theories. Ever new generations of infectors are thereby sent into practical life, and it remains to be seen when the last village physician and midwife will infect for the last time. The medical literature for the last twelve years continues to swell with reports of puerperal epidemics, and in 1854 in Vienna, the birthplace of my theory, 400 maternity patients died from childbed fever. In published medical works my teachings are either ignored or attacked. The medical faculty at Würzburg awarded a prize to a monograph written in 1859 in which my teachings were rejected. I will cite directors of maternity hospitals who have successfully followed my teachings and who have nevertheless contested them and ascribed their success to other circumstances. *[275]* Indignation over this scandal has forced the pen into my resisting hand. I would regard myself a criminal should I continue to leave it to time and unbiased evaluation to spread my teachings.

Many factors cause scientists to resist the truth so obstinately—cause men seeking to save human life to espouse so obstinately a theory that condemns to death those who are cared for as required by that theory, and indeed, achieves their deaths by the hands of those who are taught to save them. I will not mention all the factors that have prevented adoption of the law previously recommended. To discuss them while the law is not in operation would achieve nothing; it would only promote suffering. Once the law is in operation, its consequences would make these factors vanish even without discussion.

However, I am able to do something about two obstacles to the practical utilization of my teachings. One is my opponents' custom, for the pure love of truth, of referring in their attacks only to my other opponents. Indeed, Carl Braun so belies the truth as to claim that "in Germany, France, and England, the hypothesis of cadaverous infection has been almost unanimously rejected up to the present day."[1] Not everyone is familiar with the totality of the literature. Given such pronouncements, those less familiar with the literature will certainly not be challenged to think about these doctrines and to employ them. *[276]* I will bring together all that has been said in favor of my teachings in order to offset the reticence of my opponents. I expose myself freely to charges of self-praise in the hope that I will induce many to serious, unbiased thought and to conversion. The second factor that hinders the practical utilization of my teachings is the many objections that have been lodged against them. I can understand that many are impressed by these objections; it requires someone dedicated and conversant with these matters to reveal errors hidden in what is represented as truth. Just as I have collected everything that has been said in my favor, I will present even more conscientiously everything that has been said against me. I will then no longer owe the critics a response. I know that this course invites the odium of many experts. I am comforted by the knowledge that this rebuttal is not itself a goal, but only a means of bringing many physicians to the truth—physicians who may otherwise be deceived by the siren calls of my opponents. I cite now (as far as possible in chronological order) the praise that I have earned and the reproof that I have harvested.

The first public notice appeared in the *Zeitschrift der k. k. Gesellschaft der Ärzte zu Wien,* Dr. Ferdinand Hebra, editor,[2] where two editorials appeared: *[277]*

> The editors feel obliged to communicate observations made by Dr. Semmelweis, assistant at the first obstetrical clinic of the local

---

1. Carl Braun, *Lehrbuch der Geburtshülfe* (Vienna: Braumüller, 1857), p. 921.

2. Ferdinand Ritter von Hebra (1816–80) is sometimes identified as the founder of dermatology. He, like Josef Skoda and Karl Rokitansky, became a leader of the Vienna medical school. He seems always to have been supportive of Semmelweis. After his breakdown, when Semmelweis was taken back to Vienna, it was Hebra who met the train.

Imperial General Hospital, regarding puerperal fever, which rages in nearly all maternity hospitals. Dr. Semmelweis has already served more than five years in the local hospital. He has been thoroughly educated in the various branches of the medical arts, both in dissection and in bedside studies, and in the last two years has applied himself specifically to obstetrics. He set himself the task of seeking the cause of the prevalent epidemic puerperal processes. In this area nothing was left unexamined, and everything that could exert any harmful influence was conscientiously removed.

Through daily visits to the Institute for Pathological Anatomy, Dr. Semmelweis became acquainted with a harmful influence that operates through ichor and foul discharges even on the unharmed parts of the bodies of those who take part in autopsies of corpses.[3] This observation suggested to him that perhaps pregnant and laboring patients are inoculated by the obstetricians themselves, and that the disease is, in most cases, nothing other than an infection from corpses. To test this opinion an ordinance was adopted in the labor room of the first obstetrical clinic that everyone who examined patients must first wash in an aqueous solution of chloride of lime. *[278]* The results were astonishingly successful. During April and May, before this measure had been adopted, for each 100 births there were over 18 deaths. In the following months, through and including 26 November, of 1,547 births there were 47 deaths, that is, for each 100 births there were 2.45 [actually 3.04] deaths. This may also explain why schools for midwives achieve mortality rates so favorable in comparison with those for obstetricians (excepting, of course, the Maternité in Paris where, as is well-known, midwives perform autopsies).

Three particular experiences may support this conception and, indeed, expand its scope. Dr. Semmelweis believes himself able to prove that first, in September, through negligent washing by a few students who were occupied with anatomy, several patients perished, second, in October, through frequent examinations of a patient with discharging medullary carcinoma of the uterus, after which washings were not observed, and third, through the presence of a patient with a discharging leg wound, many of the patients present became infected at the same time. Therefore, the

3. Semmelweis never suggested this in his published works; this was almost certainly a misunderstanding of Semmelweis's views.

transfer of exuding ichor from living organisms can cause puerperal fever.

In announcing these experiences, we request the directors of
all maternity clinics, many of whom Dr. Semmelweis may already have notified of these most important observations, to report their confirming or disconfirming evidence.[4]

[279] The second editorial reads:

In December 1847, the editors announced the extremely important experiences of Dr. Semmelweis, assistant at the first obstetrical clinic, in respect to the etiology of epidemics of puerperal
fever in maternity hospitals. As readers will recall, the experience
was the following: maternity patients became ill primarily after
examinations by physicians whose hands were contaminated in
autopsies, and who had washed only in the ordinary fashion.
However, in no cases, or in only a few cases, did patients become
ill if examiners first washed their hands in an aqueous solution of
chloride of lime.

This most important discovery, worthy of being placed beside
Jenner's discovery of cowpox inoculations, has been completely
confirmed in the local maternity hospital, and supporting testi-
monials have been received from foreign countries. Confirming
communications have been received from Michaelis in Kiel and
from [Christian Bernard] Tilanus in Amsterdam. *[280]* In order
for this discovery to achieve its full validation, directors of obstetrical institutions are requested to conduct investigations and
to send confirming or disconfirming results to the editors of this
journal.[5]

Dr. Carl Haller, chief physician and provisional adjunct director of the Imperial Hospital in Vienna, published reports from

4. [Ferdinand Hebra, "Höchst wichtige Erfahrungen über die Ätiologie der in
Gebäranstalten epidemischen Puerperalfieber"], *Zeitschrift der k. k. Gesellschaft der
Ärzte zu Wien* 4(1847): 242–44. [Reprinted in Tiberius von Györy, *Semmelweis'
gesammelte Werke* (Jena: Gustav Fischer, 1905), pp. 23f.; author's note.]

5. [Ferdinand Hebra, "Fortsetzung der Erfahrungen über die Ätiologie der in
Gebäranstalten epidemischen Puerperalfieber"], *Zeitschrift der k. k. Gesellschaft der
Ärzte zu Wien* 5(1848): 64f. [Reprinted in Györy, op. cit., note 4 above, pp. 24f.;
author's note.]

both clinics in his "Physicians Report regarding the k. k. General Hospital of Vienna and Associated Institutions." [He wrote:]

> The mortality rates of the two gratis divisions of the maternity hospital are nearly equal and must be regarded as favorable in every respect. Everyone knows that for years there was a difference. Under Professor Klein's direction the first clinic, which was exclusively for male students, had a significantly larger mortality rate than Professor [Franz Xaver] Bartsch's school for midwives.
> The explanation for this disquieting phenomenon was never conclusively established. Dr. Semmelweis, the emeritus assistant of the first maternity clinic, performed the great service of discovering the explanation. He was guided by the conjecture that the majority of the deaths in the first clinic may be due to introduction of a poison from corpses through manual examination by students and obstetricians who were also occupied in the dissection room, and that this poison could not be completely removed by ordinary washing with soap and water. Consequently, in May 1847, with the agreement of Professor Klein, he required students and physicians to wash carefully with a chlorinated lime solution before examining patients and after examinations of patients who were even slightly ill. *[281]* Even in the first month the consequences of this rule have been astoundingly successful. [Haller gives some statistics both for women and for the newborn, and mentions that the results have been confirmed with experiments on animals. He then concludes:] *[282]* . . . The significance of this discovery for maternity hospitals, for hospitals generally, and particularly for surgical institutions, is so immeasurable as to be worthy of the most serious consideration by all men of science and by the government.[6]

Although at the close of both editorials directors of maternity hospitals were requested to report relevant information, I did not regard it as superfluous to communicate directly with the directors. My friends and I wrote to the directors of several maternity hospitals. Many of these letters were not answered.

6. Carl Haller, "Ärztlicher Bericht über das k. k. allgemeine Krankenhaus in Wien und die damit vereinigten Anstalten," *Zeitschrift der k. k. Gesellschaft der Ärzte zu Wien* 5(1849); [493–581]: 536f. [The relevant paragraphs are reprinted in Györy, op. cit., note 4 above, pp. 34f.; author's note.]

The first answer came quickly from [James Young] Simpson at Edinburgh.[7] Dr. Arneth, my friend and colleague from the second clinic, was more fluent in English than I. He wrote to Simpson, but unfortunately I am unable to reprint the response because, as Arneth has personally assured me, the letter was lost during the intervening years. This letter was full of abuse. Simpson said that he knew, even without our letter, the lamentable condition of obstetrics in Germany and especially in Vienna. He knew certainly that the cause of our great mortality lay in the boundless neglect from which maternity patients suffered, that, for example, without even changing the linen, healthy patients were placed in beds in which others had died. *[283]* [Simpson also surmised that] English obstetrical literature must be totally unknown to us, otherwise we would have known that the English have long regarded childbed fever as contagious and would have employed chlorine washings to protect against it. After this letter we saw no reason to continue our correspondence with Professor Simpson.

Simpson could regard my opinions on the origin of childbed fever as identical with those of the English only because of excessive haste. This follows from correspondence I carried out with Dr. [Charles Henry Felix] Routh in London. Dr. Routh visited the first clinic as a student while I was the assistant; he became convinced of the correctness of my teachings. He returned to his homeland with the intention of making my opinions known there. His first letter contained the following:

> In a meeting of English physicians in the last week of November 1848, I gave a lecture in which I announced your discovery. As was just, you received the greatest credit. I can say that my lecture was well received, and that many of the most informed

7. Sir James Young Simpson (1811–70) was Professor of Obstetrics at the University of Edinburgh. Semmelweis refers to him as "the most famous obstetrician of our times." (Ibid., p. 68). At first he apparently believed that Semmelweis was advancing the same views as those already espoused by the British. By the end of his life, however, he had moved much closer to Semmelweis, and some of his later essays seem to reflect even more indebtedness to Semmelweis than Simpson ever admitted.

members testified that the evidence was conclusive. *[284]* In particular [John] Webster, [George A.] Copeland, and [Edward Wil-
liam] Murphy, all distinguished physicians, spoke most favorably. The report of this discussion is contained in the November
issue of *Lancet*.[8]

After I left [Vienna] did the cases continue to support your
opinion? Is childbed fever more or less prevalent? If this dangerous disease is no longer in the obstetrical wards, that confirms a
meaningful success. The frequent occurrence of childbed fever in
Prague is to be ascribed to the same cause. My description of
your discovery has been published in a pamphlet.[9]

[In a subsequent letter Routh observed:] *[285]* "The fame and
truth of your discovery spread continually wider in the general
opinion. All societies of physicians know and admit how useful
it is. That does not appear unreasonable, for the truth is great
and will win out."[10]

Murphy, formerly Professor of Obstetrics at Dublin and currently at London, wrote a long article in which he discussed
Routh's lecture and accepted the views expressed therein.[11] Even
Simpson has given up the opinion that childbed fever is contagious. He now holds childbed fever to be identical with surgical
fever and writes,

The fever is not itself the cause of the attendant inflammations,
nor these inflammations themselves the cause of the attendant
fever; but both of them—that is, both the fever and the inflammations—are simultaneous sequences or effects of one common
cause—namely, the original vitiated or diseased condition of the

8. Charles Henry Felix Routh, "On the Causes of the Endemic Puerperal
Fever of Vienna," *Medico-chirurgical Transactions* 32(1849): 27–40. The lecture was
delivered by Edward William Murphy since Routh was not a Fellow of the Royal
Medical and Surgical Society. The review that Routh mentions was in *Lancet*
2(1848): 642f. For a list of some other reviews, see Frank P. Murphy, "Ignaz
Philipp Semmelweis (1818–1865): An Annotated Bibliography," *Bulletin of the
History of Medicine* 20(1946), 653–707: 654f.

9. Dorset-Square, London, 21 May 1849 [author's note].

10. Dorset-Square, London, 3 December 1849 [author's note].

11. Edward William Murphy, ["Puerperal Fever"], *Dublin Quarterly Journal of
Medical Science* [24] (1857): [1–30. But Murphy also says that puerperal fever can
have many other causes besides decaying organic matter; author's note.]

general circulating fluid. . . . What this vitiated condition of the blood may specifically and actually consist of . . . a more subtle chemistry and histology . . . will, perhaps, yet ultimately determine.[12]

The cause of the blood's disintegration, the common cause of the fever and the inflammation that accompany childbed fever and surgical fever, has already been identified as the resorption of decaying animal-organic matter.

[286] The second answer came from Professor Michaelis from Kiel. Dr. Schwartz, Michaelis's student, attended the practical obstetrics course in the first clinic at the end of 1847. He wrote to Michaelis describing the observations that had been made in Vienna; the answering letter read as follows:

Your letter of 21 December 1847 has excited my highest interest. I was in the greatest need. Because of puerperal fever our institution was closed from 1 July until 1 November. The first three patients admitted thereafter became ill; one died and two were barely saved. We intended, therefore, to close the institution again. Then conditions improved; two new cases of illness were easily cured. One patient died in February; since then all are healthy. Your communication gave me renewed courage; the proof of the usefulness of chlorine washings, as they were practiced in Vienna, is already of great significance because of the large numbers involved. I adopted the washings immediately in the institution, and since then no one, neither student nor midwife, has been allowed to examine without having washed with chlorine. It is also used by a midwife in the city who formerly delivered many women who later suffered puerperal fever.

12. [James Young] Simpson, ["Notes on the Analogy between Puerperal Fever and Surgical Fever"], *Monthly Journal of Medical Science* [11] (1850), [414–29: 420f. I have taken the quotation from the original rather than retranslating Semmelweis's version. Semmelweis's views were much more favorably received in England than on the continent, but even in England he was more often cited than understood. The English consistently regarded Semmelweis as having supported their theory of contagion. A typical example was W. Tyler Smith who claimed that Semmelweis "made out very conclusively" that "miasms derived from the dissecting-room will excite puerperal disease." "Puerperal Fever," *Lancet* 2(1856), 503–05: 504; author's note.]

I have also sent a copy of your letter to Copenhagen. To speak of my own experience, which is so small in comparison with the extensive experiment in Vienna, would be presumptuous. However, I cannot refrain from communicating something to you that is obviously connected with these matters. *[287]* Last summer my cousin died of puerperal fever. I had examined her after delivery at a time when I had autopsied patients who had died of puerperal fever. From that time I was convinced of communicability. It occurred to me that a few months earlier, a woman in the city to whom I had been called also died of childbed fever. I avoided being present at births for four weeks. One delivering patient whom I was supposed to help was therefore required to call a different physician. This physician performed autopsies daily. There was a prolapse of the umbilical cord; he replaced it. The delivering woman contracted puerperal fever. She was saved, but she had an exuding mass in her uterus. The midwife who cared for her had at least two, perhaps three, cases of puerperal fever in the city. So much for the propagation of the disease.

I can recommend very emphatically the security gained through chlorine washing. The hands retain the smell for several days in spite of repeated washing; but this is not the case with chlorine washing. Since adopting this practice, no one delivered by me or by my pupils has contracted the slightest degree of fever, with the exception of an isolated case in February in which a poorly cleaned catheter was used. After the dangerous beginning in November, however, I expected a horrible epidemic. My experience is limited to about thirty cases because we admit only a very few pregnant women. I thank you for your communication, therefore, from my whole heart; it may have saved our institution from being disbanded. It would perhaps have been impossible to solicit a new hospital at this time. I extend congratulations to Dr. Semmelweis for what is probably a great discovery.

You know that puerperal fever has been with us since 1834. *[288]* That is also about the time when I began to occupy myself actively in teaching and when I instituted vaginal examinations by students. This fact may also be related.[13]

Thus, in the Kiel maternity hospital, my opinion of the origin of childbed fever was strikingly confirmed. The smallness of the institution is not relevant. If a hospital is large enough that a

13. Kiel, 18 March 1848 [author's note].

puerperal epidemic may force it to close, it is also large enough to be accepted as evidence if an epidemic is prevented.

Another of Michaelis's students later came to Vienna and I inquired about Michaelis. I was horrified to discover that he had died. Experiences further confirmed his conviction that he was responsible for the death of his cousin. He sank into a deep melancholy, and threw himself under a train speeding into Hamburg. I have related Michaelis's unfortunate death as a monument to his sensitive conscience. Unfortunately, I will also exhibit to the reader obstetricians whose consciences lack that of which Michaelis's had too much. May his remains rest in peace.

After I had resolved to step once more before the public, it seemed important to write to Michaelis's successor, Professor Litzmann, to ask what he had observed in the institution where Michaelis's experiences confirmed mine. I received the following answer:

> [289] . . . During the ten years that I have directed the local maternity hospital, I have tried to exclude every opportunity for maternity patients to become infected by poison from corpses. My assistants and I avoid all direct participation in autopsies and require students to observe all known cautionary measures. In fact, I have been more fortunate than my predecessor respecting puerperal fever, and I have only a few victims to mourn.
>
> I attribute this favorable state of affairs to a precaution against all overcrowding. The institution has seven single rooms for patients. The rule has been that each patient has a room to herself for at least the first five to seven days. This room also serves as a delivery room. In the second week after delivery two patients are put into each room. Experience shows that if the number of patients exceeds ten, so that in the first days after delivery patients must share rooms, and rooms are reused without being aired out, childbed fever is immediately encountered. I have therefore sought to reduce admissions as far as possible so that, indeed, in the winter months the number of patients seldom exceeds ten. When necessary I have placed delivering patients in private locations that I have rented in the neighborhood of the hospital; they deliver there. I have always done this when cases of childbed fever occurred in the institution. Michaelis did not always observe these

precautions. Under his direction there were approximately 160–90 births annually; I never allow births to exceed 150. *[290]* Of course, in spite of all precautions, I have not been spared small epidemic or endemic outbreaks, and twice I have been obliged to close the institution temporarily. But with the exception of one patient who died, those in private locations remained healthy or they became only mildly ill. I will also observe that childbed fever occasionally manifests itself first in the city, or in the surroundings and then later in the institution, or the institution may be completely spared.[14]

In this letter Professor Litzmann claims to observe measures against infection. He affirms a favorable condition of health among the patients; however, he believes that this condition is due to his precautions against overcrowding. I do not share this belief. When Michaelis reopened the hospital after having closed it for four months, the first 3 patients became ill. The maternity hospital was certainly ventilated, and it was certainly not overcrowded, with 3 patients. Litzmann set great store on admitting only 150 patients a year, while Michaelis admitted 160–90. Kiwisch cared for 102 patients a year and 26.47 percent died; in Vienna in 1822, 3,066 patients were cared for and only .84 percent died. Litzmann allows only 1 patient in a room. At the first clinic 32 patients were cared for in one room, but while we washed with chlorine there were two months with no deaths. During the five least favorable months before chlorine washings, the hospital was much less crowded than in the two months when we had no deaths. I have shown with numerous tables how insignificant overcrowding is. *[291]* I therefore assert that the ten years of favorable health in the Kiel maternity hospital are due to measures against infection.

Michaelis said in his letter that he had forwarded a copy of Dr. Schwartz's letter to Copenhagen. I therefore requested Professor Levy to inform me of his observations in the intervening ten years. [In response, Levy explained that he had replied to Schwartz's original letter and that the letter, together with his

14. Kiel, 25 September 1858 [author's note].

reply, had been published in a local medical periodical. He had
sent copies to Michaelis and had assumed that these had been
forwarded to Semmelweis. Discovering now that Semmelweis
had not received the reply, he included a copy. Levy explained
that they had little occasion to try chlorine washings because the
hospital was so arranged that students and the resident faculty
seldom contaminated their hands with decaying organic matter.
He continues:] *[292]*

> . . . For more than ten years in the maternity institution we have
> had a rule that corpses of puerperae are not dissected by physi-
> cians or clinicians of the institution; we employ outside help for
> this purpose. We perform autopsies only in exceptional cases when
> the cause of death is not puerperal fever, and even then with the
> precaution that the person performing the autopsy tries to avoid
> examining patients on the same day. In a different area we have
> had rich opportunity to accumulate experience, for we dissect all
> the corpses of children both from here and from the general hos-
> pital. These dissections take place three or four times a week.
> They are nearly all performed by our reserve physicians without
> any special precautions other than to preserve ordinary cleanli-
> ness. While these same persons frequently participate in exami-
> nations and operations on women giving birth, we have not ob-
> served the least cause to regret these dissections. *[293]* In the course
> of the year we employ chlorine washings only when it is neces-
> sary to deal with decayed and stinking preparations.[15]

[Levy concludes his letter by apologizing for the harshness of
the published reply. The following excerpts are from that reply
(which responded to the original letter that had been sent by
Schwartz and forwarded by Michaelis).]

> With all due respect and consideration for the meritorious work
> revealed in Dr. Semmelweis's examination, I believe that I must
> not withhold the following observations and reservations. Above
> all it is to be regretted that neither the observations nor the opin-
> ions grounded on them are presented with the clarity and pre-
> cision that would be desirable in such an important matter of
> etiology. To presume that corpses can and do infect, without

15. Copenhagen, 31 May 1858 [author's note].

considering whether the infection is derived from puerperae or from other corpses, is as much a consequence of unrecognized a priori assumptions as of the cited facts. A strict examination would absolutely require that different sources of infection be taken into account and provide the basis for a classification of the observations. *[294]* From a scientific point of view, particularly regarding the question of the contagiousness of puerperal fever, it is important to know whether the presumed cadaveric infection is to be ascribed only to puerperal cadaverous matter or rather to all cadaverous effluvium in general. It is also important to know whether puerperal disease occasioned by infection from corpses occurs in one identical form or in different forms, depending on various cadaveric sources of infection. It would be enlightening, insofar as the discussion concerns only puerperal corpses, to consider whether the contagium is present in the superficial parts, since we are concerned with the products of a disease assumed to be transferable to nearby predisposed persons. On the other hand, if the infective matter can originate from all corpses, one must give up every notion of a specific contagium and look instead for an infection of the blood mass. Insofar as such an infection exists, it must be grouped with the many experiments on animals in which the direct introduction of putrid animal matter causes blood infection in the organism. One cannot doubt that in this way a condition is caused that has many similarities to puerperal pyemia. But the observation is also firmly established that puerperal fever manifests itself in different forms, and thus it would have been desirable for the examination to have proceeded with less indifference to questions regarding differences in the sources, nature, and operation of infective cadaverous matter.[16]

[295] Every corpse, regardless of the disease that caused death, can bring about childbed fever. It follows that childbed fever is not a contagious disease; it is rather a pyemia such as is brought on in experiments on animals. Puerperal fever certainly manifests itself in different forms; it is also certain that these forms come about in the same way as do cases of pyemia. The form of puerperal fever that is known as pyemia occurs less frequently

16. [Karl Edouard Marius] Levy, ["De nyeste Forsög i Födselsstiftelsen i Wien til Oplysning om Barselfeberens Aetiologie"], *Hospitals-Meddelelser* 1(1848), [199–211: 204–6; author's note].

than other forms of puerperal fever. Cases of childbed fever at the first clinic were certainly not all of the form known as pyemia, but they were all prevented by chlorine washings. This proves that they all had the same cause. However, we do not know why at one time decaying, resorbed matter causes pyemia, while at other times it causes other forms of disease. Perhaps the reason lies in the different degrees of corruption of the decaying matter, or perhaps in the different susceptibilities of the organism. . . .

[296] [Semmelweis continues to quote from Levy:]

The quantitative limits of a specific contagium are incalculable. It is possible, under favorable conditions, that a single atom would be sufficient to transfer the disease. Indeed, in questions of contagiousness no possibility can confidently be denied a priori. Therefore, from the standpoint of contagiousness, if Dr. Semmelweis had limited his opinion regarding infections from corpses to puerperal corpses, I would have been less disposed to denial than I am. I do not otherwise believe in contagion, but simply out of scrupulous consideration for the possibility, for several years we have taken care that no physician would have contact with a woman giving birth on the same day that he had dissected a puerperal corpse. I should add immediately that I have had in mind not so much the transferring of palpable infective matter by examination as the possible operation of a vapor from the corpse that adheres to the hands, the hair, and the clothing. *[297]* However, as already noted, the specific contagium seems to be of little importance to Dr. Semmelweis. Indeed it is so little considered that he does not even discuss the direct transmission of the disease from those who are ill to healthy persons lying nearby. He is concerned only with general infection from corpses without respect to the disease that led to death. In this respect his opinion seems improbable. Semmelweis has exaggerated the absorptive capacity of the healthy uterus in transferring matter [into an organism]—this capacity certainly cannot be demonstrated experimentally by its operation on drugs introduced there by the physician. Beyond this, the speed and intensity of the resulting reaction appear to depend on quantitative considerations; a rapidly fatal putrid infection, even if the putrid matter is introduced directly into the blood, requires more than homeopathic doses of the poi-

son. And, with due respect for the cleanliness of the Viennese
students, it seems improbable that enough infective matter or vapor could be secluded around the fingernails to kill a patient.[17]

[Semmelweis points out that he does not regard childbed fever
as contagious and that the uterus is resorbant only because the
mucous membrane has been damaged by pregnancy. He continues:] *[298]* . . . In order to determine the material quantum of
decaying matter that is necessary to cause childbed fever, it would
be necessary to conduct direct experiments. I prefer to remain
uncertain on this point, and am content to know that however
much is left after ordinary washing is sufficient, even if this is in
the form of a putrid vapor. I proved this by destroying the decaying matter that remained on the hands after ordinary washing
and thereby reducing the mortality in the first clinic.

To prove his opinion, Dr. Semmelweis ordered chlorine washings to destroy every trace of cadaverous residue on the fingers.
Would not the experiment have been simpler and more reliable if
it had been arranged, at least during the experiment, that all anatomical work would be avoided? For the two or three months
of the obstetrical course, this requirement would have involved
no great cost for the students. *[299]* In our maternity hospital,
without intending anything experimental, and simply trying to
be scrupulous regarding the possibility of contagiousness, for more
than a year we have forbidden physicians, midwives, and attendants to have close contact with puerperal corpses. Without knowing how this one regulation may have improved the health of
patients, I am of the opinion that it will be continued and that for
autopsies we will continue to rely on the assistance of external
colleagues.

[Semmelweis notes that he certainly agrees that keeping the hands
clean is an effective means of preventing childbed fever and that

17. Ibid., pp. 206f. Various of Semmelweis's critics pointed out, as Levy has
in the preceding passage, that the quantity of decaying matter that would be
retained on the hands would simply be inadequate to kill a person either chemically or physically. Robert Koch later used precisely this fact to prove that various infecting materials contained living organisms which could reproduce in the
human body, i.e. that since the poison could be neither chemical nor physical in
operation, it must be biological.

for this reason he has advocated a law that would require precisely that. He then continues to quote Levy.]

[300] In spite of these reservations, one must admit that the results of the experiment appear to support Dr. Semmelweis's opinion, but certainly one must admit no more. Everyone who has had the opportunity to observe the periodic variations in the mortality rate of maternity clinics will agree that his findings lack certain important confirmation. Namely, [the question remains] whether in earlier years the institution has not also had periods as favorable as the last seven months. One lacks exact statistical information regarding the monthly mortality rates in the earlier period. About three years ago Professor Klein officially reported a mortality rate of one in fifteen; while tragic enough, this was 100 percent better than the mortality rate of the period against which the results of the chlorine washings were judged. It is possible, indeed probable, that [Semmelweis's evidence] is due less to a constant improvement in conditions of health than to particular more favorable periods. In the absence of more precise statistical information, it is conceivable that the results of the last seven months depend partially on periodic accidental factors, and partially on stricter concern for general cleanliness occasioned by the experiment itself.[18]

[301] Time has refuted this point, we are no longer concerned with seven months but with twelve years. Professor Levy holds expectations for a student's letter that can only be satisfied by a complete monograph. The attentive reader will find the solution to all Levy's doubts. In particular, the reader will not have cause to complain about the lack of exact statistical information. . . .

In September and October [1847] the results of the experiment were less than expected. Dr. Semmelweis believes himself able to prove that this was caused in part by students' neglect of chlorine washings and in part by infection of patients from ichorous wounds. He finds here not only confirmation of his original opinion, but an endlessly expanding perspective within which all ichorous secretions from living organisms can be included. [302] In this respect, the experiences cited are all too hastily sketched

18. Ibid., pp. 207–9.

to enable the critic to draw a conclusion. It is important to know whether the patients with discharging wounds were also suffering from puerperal fever. If so, the puerperal contagium would replace the presumed ichorous infection as the specific contagium. Otherwise, the first case [the woman with a carious knee] is clearly inconsistent with the possibility of infection [since presumably she must have infected herself], while the second case [the woman with the cancer in her uterus] remains strikingly unclear. Could ichor from this patient have been more damaging when conveyed in vaginal examinations to other patients than it would have been as a result of similar examinations carried out on this patient herself? In our hospital we have frequently recorded ichorous sores on the feet of delivering patients without having noticed any subsequent infections, either of those patients themselves or of other patients. Dr. Semmelweis places great emphasis on the better health of institutions exclusively for the education of midwives; he should consider that ichorous secretions occur equally in both institutions. Moreover, in an institution as large as the midwife clinic in Vienna, one or another of the patients must always be ill and so provide a source of infection. If the infection occurs as easily as he believes, this would reduce the inequality in mortality rates between the clinics.[19]

[303] The two diseased patients did not have childbed fever. The patient with the discharging medullary carcinoma of the uterus died from the cancer. The patient with the carious wound was released after a successful delivery.[20] . . . I identified three sources of the decaying matter that causes puerperal fever: every corpse, every sick person who generates decaying matter, and all animal-organic physiological products that decompose. In maternity hospitals for midwives the first of these sources is missing; this explains the superior health in clinics for midwives. . . .

19. Ibid., pp. 209–11.

20. At this point Semmelweis refers the reader back to his original description of these cases (see above, pp. 92f.; German edition, pp. 58–60) where, he says, one will find the solution to this difficulty. In fact Semmelweis had no solution, and subsequent critics recognized this deficiency as a serious weakness in his position. It seemed incredible that, if Semmelweis were correct, these two women could have infected other patients without becoming infected themselves.

[304–6] In conclusion Professor Levy writes, "These are my impressions of Dr. Semmelweis's experiences; for these reasons I must judge provisionally that his opinions are not clear enough and his findings not exact enough to qualify as scientifically founded."[21] Nothing remains but to recommend that Professor Levy study the present essay diligently. I do not doubt that he will also come to the conviction that in place of the colossal nonsense that has been taught regarding the origin of childbed fever, I have erected a clear scientific structure supported by reliable experience, one that lacks only universal recognition to yield those blessings for which it was intended.

Before continuing with the correspondence with Professor Levy, it will be useful to publish the following letter from Professor [József] Dietl of Krakow.[22] . . .

> Everywhere on my journey I observed that your opinion regarding the origin of childbed fever is reflected in the organization of maternity hospitals. Ill patients are conscientiously isolated, and as in Copenhagen, physicians have no contact with corpses. Of course I cannot indicate with what success. . . . *[307]* In general one hears less of the devastations of puerperal epidemics. Perhaps the reason lies in adoption of the orientation that is based on your experience, without anyone being willing to admit it to himself or to the public.[23]

I continue now with Levy. I wrote to Levy and attempted to resolve the doubts he raised. I observed, however, that it was more important for me to know what he now believed, after ten years, than what doubts he had raised ten years earlier. Receiv-

21. Levy, op. cit., note 16 above, p. 211.
22. József Dietl (1804–78) was perhaps the most outspoken representative of therapeutic nihilism, a controversial movement that became prominent in about the middle of the nineteenth century. Those associated with this movement were skeptical of existing therapies and believed that rational therapies could only be established after the chemical, physical and biological properties of the body were better understood. In some cases the opinion was expressed that since existing therapies were unfounded and more likely to do harm than good, the physician should simply rely on nature to cure rather than to employ standard therapies.
23. Krakow, 28 April 1858 [author's note].

ing no reply, I wrote again. In this letter I wrote that I knew that the Copenhagen maternity hospital had earlier been ravaged by childbed fever to such a degree that its existence was threatened. I wrote what Professor Dietl had written concerning the Copenhagen hospital. I also wrote what Professor Braun had said about the Copenhagen hospital, namely that "because this is the most appropriate and noteworthy newly constructed maternity hospital, in which every step has been taken to halt puerperal fever epidemics, we allow ourselves to estimate that in this new building under Levy's direction no puerperal fever epidemics will occur."[24] I closed by asking whether the improved health could be attributed to prophylactic measures for which my opinion had in any way been responsible.

[308] I received the following reply:

> . . . It is not clear to me how you can ask whether it was as a result of your opinion that changes were made in the maternity hospital at Copenhagen. Even had it been known to us, your opinion on the origin of puerperal fever would have had no influence on the reconstruction and hygienic reorganization of the hospital. I do not understand what influence these opinions could have on the organization of an institution. Precautionary measures were taken in the regulations of the hospital to guard against conveying cadaverous matter to maternity patients in examining them. However, on the broader organization of the institution I can think of no influences.
>
> I have already responded clearly enough to your opinions. If you have given my writings sufficient attention you will remember that before your opinions were known to us, out of concern for contagion, we had taken scrupulous steps to guard against infection from puerperal corpses. It may be that later, out of respect for your opinion, we were more cautious in non-puerperal autopsies than we had previously been. Nevertheless, we do undertake these autopsies ourselves, while we employ external help for those of patients who die of puerperal fever. *[309]* What part such precautionary measures may have had in the improved health

24. Carl Braun, "Zur Lehre und Behandlung der Puerperalprocesse und ihrer Beziehungen zu einigen zymotischen Krankheiten," in Baptist Johann Chiari, Carl Braun, and Joseph Späth, *Klinic der Geburtshilfe und Gynäkologie* (Erlangen: Enke, 1855), p. 433.

at the institution cannot be calculated, because at the same time we also instituted highly important changes in the physical facilities and in administrative organization.[25]

Who that is unbiased does not recall the words of Professor Dietl: "In general one hears less of the devastations of puerperal epidemics. Perhaps the reason lies in adoption of the orientation that is based on your experience, without anyone being willing to admit it to himself or to the public." Professor Levy says that it cannot be calculated what part the precautionary measures had in the improved health because the physical facilities and the administration were also changed. It is certain that the construction and administration of the Copenhagen hospital did not change the atmospheric-cosmic-terrestrial circumstances of Copenhagen. The earlier great mortality was not, therefore, due to atmospheric influences; it was not an epidemic. And if, as a result of measures which were employed to prevent external decaying matter from being transmitted, the health of the hospital improved, this is proof of the truth of my theory.

[310] Tilanus of Amsterdam wrote the following.

. . . During my twenty years as director of the present institution, I have examined these matters carefully. I have found no reason to depart from a view held here long before my time. Namely that once the disease has begun, because of an epidemic atmospheric condition such as variable winter or spring weather, its distribution and duration among maternity patients should be attributed to a definite contagiousness. In part, my opinion is based on the often clearly demonstrable origin of the disease from one who was already ill during the birth. After a short time the disease is conveyed to healthy patients who deliver at the same time and who are placed in the same environment as the diseased patient. Moreover, the end of an epidemic often comes when births decrease so that diseased patients can be isolated. Their care can then be left to people who are carefully excluded from subsequent births and from newly admitted patients.

It is clear that such experiences are possible only in a relatively small institution (we average 400 births each year). This also ex-

25. Copenhagen, 21 September 1858 [author's note].

plains why the opposing view is so firmly espoused in the larger
institutions, although the explanations of communication by
contagium cannot be contested either in theory or by analogy.
[311] Most striking is the analogy with septic fever which threat-
ens the recently wounded in surgical wards. A newly delivered
person is, after all, in the same physiological condition as a newly
wounded person. I fully agree with your opinion that contagium
from corpses is the cause of the disease. In earlier years I traced
particular cases to this cause; since then I have taken the strictest
measures to protect against this misfortune.

Assistants and students who perform manual examinations and
who attend deliveries must completely refrain from anatomical
activities. Autopsies of patients who die from puerperal fever are
carried out by people from medical or surgical wards or by other
students. At the very most those who will not be on call for a
few days are allowed to attend these autopsies and to see the results, but they are strictly forbidden to contaminate their hands.
It is my conviction that we may not sacrifice those entrusted to
us simply because of a curiosity that can be satisfied in due course.
I admit that these precautions can be reduced through conscientious cleansing with a chlorine solution (we always use this in the
institution, for attendants and in autopsies), but they should never
be given up completely.

We do not understand the nature of cadaveric poison, and we
cannot know whether it is destroyed by our disinfectants. In any
case this is not suggested by experience; we observe that neither
puerperal fever, septic fever, nor hospital effluvium can be oblit-
erated by cleaning and fumigating with chlorine vapor unless the
infected spaces are exposed to an unbroken stream of air for a
long period of time.

[312] I am happy to report that this winter the patients have
been generally healthy. We have had only sporadic cases of fever.
Of 133 who were delivered between November and February,
only 2 died. In December, at the beginning of the winter cold,
the disease threatened to become epidemic; 5 newly delivered patients were seriously afflicted within three days. Fortunately, all
were saved through energetic antiphlogistic measures, however,
the weather then remained consistently cold over a period of six
weeks and thereafter we had no frost. Such a period of unbroken
weather is unusual for us, especially in spring. Last year between
January and April 12 patients died; from May until September
none died, in October 2 died. In the last months births were about

equally spaced, so we have not been overcrowded. At my urgent request we have changed location and are now so arranged that normally we are only half occupied.

Finally, I hope that your humane efforts will have a great impact upon the harmful beliefs that this disease is not contagious and that poison from corpses is harmless. Kiwisch has recently advocated these beliefs. His assurances that immediately after autopsies he cares for both laboring and newly delivered patients are frightening and encourage foolhardy negligence among the inexperienced. *[313]* Unfortunately, a range of harmful influences that can cause illness because of the general predisposition of maternity patients still exist outside our control. No one has grounds for believing that it will be easy for those of our opinion to extirpate these influences.[26]

Professor Skoda delivered a lecture in the Academy of Science at Vienna entitled "Regarding Dr. Semmelweis's Discovery of the True Cause of the Unusually High Incidence of Sickness among the Patients of the Viennese Maternity Hospital and the Means of Reducing This Incidence to Normal Levels."[27] The Imperial Academy of Science published the lecture in its proceedings and prepared a special reprint from the October 1849 issue. At the same time Professor [Ernst Wilhelm Ritter von] Brücke and I became full members of the Academy and were given a grant to experiment on animals. [After quoting a report by Brücke admitting that their experiments were inconclusive, Semmelweis observes,] *[314]* . . . I have had experiences at the Viennese maternity clinic and at two other institutions, and in this essay I have assembled similar experiences from others. I believe as a result of these experiences that experiments on animals are now superfluous.

Professor Skoda's lecture contained these remarks: "In the

26. Amsterdam, 9 March 1848 [author's note].

27. Josef Skoda, "Über die von Dr. Semmelweis entdeckte wahre Ursache der in der Wiener Gebäranstalt ungewöhnlich häufig vorkommenden Erkrankungen der Wöchnerinnen und das Mittles zur Verminderung dieser Erkrankungen bis auf die gewöhnliche Zahl," *Sitzungsberichte der mathematisch-naturwissenschaftlichen Classe der kaiserlichen Akademie der Wissenschaft* 3(1849): 168–80. Reprinted in Györy, op. cit., note 4 above, pp. 36–45. For references to various reviews see Murphy, op. cit., note 8 above, p. 656.

Prague maternity hospital the number of ill patients occasionally becomes very great; to all appearances this has the same cause as in Vienna. This is a circumstance that may help to clarify matters. I therefore urge that chlorine washings be instituted in the Prague hospital."[28] [Wilhelm Friedrich Scanzoni, the director in Prague, was not persuaded, however, and attacked Skoda and Semmelweis. Semmelweis, obviously regarding Scanzoni as a principal opponent, devoted more space to Scanzoni than to anyone else. Parts of Semmelweis's discussion are very repetitious.]

[315–23] . . . Scanzoni divides puerperal inflammations into such as proceed with or without blood disintegration. According to Scanzoni, the latter are not genuine puerperal fever; however, these can become genuine cases if, in the course of the disease, the products of inflammation are resorbed and lead to disintegration of the blood. Such cases include endometritis, metritis [inflammation of the uterus], metrophlebitis, [etc.]. Inflammations in which there is disintegration of the blood are genuine cases of puerperal fever. These include hyperinosis, pyemia, and the blood disintegration of puerperae. Among maternity patients and in autopsies, cases can be observed that are classified as hyperinosis, others that are classified as pyemia, others as disintegration of the blood, and still other cases that cannot be subsumed under any of these forms and that, according to Scanzoni, are to be classified as inflammations but not as puerperal fever. Nevertheless, it is certain that these are all varieties of resorption—in ordinary usage of puerperal fever—because all of these forms are consequences of the resorption of decaying matter. However, it is not known why at different times the resorbed matter generates hyperinosis, pyemia, blood disintegration, or still other forms. *[324]* As has already been explained, this may depend on the greater or lesser degree of decomposition of the resorbed matter, on the reaction of the organism, or perhaps on other circumstances. We know only that in all these cases decaying matter is resorbed and it disintegrates the blood. Sometimes, but not always, we are able to perceive the disintegration. In consequence of this disintegration, inflammation arises.

28. Györy, op. cit., note 4 above, p. 41.

This is also true if there is no apparent blood disintegration (which cases Scanzoni does not recognize as genuine puerperal fever), since these cases are also prevented by chlorine washing. . . .
[325–28] . . . Scanzoni writes:

> Chlorine washing was first adopted in the maternity hospital in Prague in March 1848 when puerperal fever was frequent and virulent. It was used continuously through the second half of March and through all of April. During this period we also visited the autopsy room only very rarely. However, since the incidence of sickness was not reduced, chlorine washings were temporarily given up as an experiment. What was not achieved with the most conscientiously undertaken and supervised washings then came about through a more favorable state of the *genius epidemicus*[29]—the incidence of disease suddenly dropped. Thus in May, of 205 patients there was only 1 death while in March and April, although we washed with chloride of lime, of 406 patients there were 31 chance [*zufällig*] deaths.[30] After becoming convinced that this measure would not stop outbreaks of disease already in progress, it occurred to us to explore whether it was perhaps sufficient to prevent an epidemic from beginning. Therefore, the washings were begun again at the beginning of June and, without a demonstrable cause, in June 21, in July 9, and in August 26 people became ill; 19 of these died. Assuming that the chlorine washings really had such a great influence, and that the frequency of disease was determined only by infections from corpses spread by examinations, we were unable to explain these striking variations.[31]

29. *Genius epidemicus* means literally the natural character or inherent constitution of the epidemic. The concept was used to explain aspects of observed cases of the epidemic. If, for example, a particular symptom seemed more common at one time than another, this would be attributed to changes in the *genius epidemicus*. Of course, since the only way of measuring the *genius epidemicus* was by the observed cases of the disease, such an attribution had no explanatory value. As Semmelweis observed, it was explaining the unknown with the unknown. See above, p. 157; German edition, p. 212.

30. By chance deaths Scanzoni may have meant that the cases were sporadic rather than epidemic. Skoda may have believed (erroneously) that Semmelweis's discovery related only to so-called epidemic childbed fever. Given contemporary conceptions, it would have been possible for sporadic cases to occur even when there was no epidemic. Of course, this was not Semmelweis's position, and later Semmelweis ridicules Scanzoni for talking about chance deaths.

31. Wilhelm Friedrich Scanzoni, "Über die von Dr. Semmelweis entdeckte,

[329] I cannot deny my wonder at Scanzoni's penetrating sagacity in dispensing with chlorine washings as an experiment. Any person with common sense would have taken the time from the opening day of the Prague maternity hospital until the day of the adoption of the chlorine washings as the period in which the washings were not used. I refer Scanzoni to the tables given at the back of the book for the Viennese maternity hospital. I cannot deny that this experiment casts an unfavorable light on his sense of responsibility. For at the time he performed this sagacious experiment, he was not completely convinced that chlorine washings were not suitable as protection against childbed fever. He first gained this conviction when, in spite of abandoning the chlorine washings, the mortality rate fell and, in spite of adopting the washings again, the mortality rate rose. It was possible, however, that my opinion would be confirmed. Suppose, as a result of discontinuing the washings, there had been a great increase in mortality. Could one conscientiously undertake such an experiment?

The reader will recall that in 1847 the first clinic had 57 fatalities in April and 36 more in May. Approximately in the middle of May we adopted chlorine washings and the mortality was reduced to 6 in June, 3 in July, and 5 in August. However, 12 patients died in September, 11 in October, 11 in November, and 8 in December. *[330]* From this increased mortality, I did not conclude that the chlorine washings were useless, but rather that decaying matter was being conveyed to the patients in spite of the washings. The ensuing examination revealed that some students had been negligent in washing, that I had not washed after examining a patient with cancer of the uterus, and that I did not isolate a patient with a carious knee. Rather than give up the chlorine washings, we practiced them more strictly. The fortunate results were that over seven months we lost less than 1 patient per 100. The years 1849 and 1850 may have been even more favorable had my request to direct the first clinic been granted. . . .

---

wahre Ursache der in der Wiener Gebäranstalt ungewöhnlich häufig vorkommenden Erkrankungen der Wöchnerinen und das Mittle zur Verminderung dieser Erkrankungen bis auf die gewöhnliche Zahl," *Vierteljahrschrift für die praktische Heilkunde* Literarischer Anzeiger, 6, no. 2(1850), 25–33: 29.

Scanzoni failed miserably when, after less than six months of unfavorable results, he hastily concluded that chlorine washings have no important influence and that the frequency of disease is not dependent on examinations by contaminated persons. The reader has seen the weighty arguments that Scanzoni has directed against me; he certainly did not conceal them from his students. When he did not reduce the mortality as suddenly as in Vienna and when the mortality increased in spite of chlorine washings, it might have occurred to Scanzoni that precisely these weighty arguments deterred the students from washing as conscientiously as necessary.[32] Not even all of my students did so, although I forcefully recommended the chlorine washings to them. . . .

[331] Scanzoni knows only one of the three sources of decaying matter, namely the corpse. Scanzoni says during this period he visited the autopsy room only very rarely. He did not know at the time that ill patients can be a source of decaying matter. The experience in the Prague maternity hospital may have been like what happened in Vienna because of the cancer of the uterus and the carious knee. We did not know at the time that decaying matter could come from the sick. If Scanzoni believed that decaying matter could come only from corpses, the head midwife and all other personnel who did not contact corpses would cer-

32. Bernhard Seyfert was Scanzoni's colleague and director of the clinic for obstetricians in Prague. A contemporary essay about Seyfert's clinic, which Semmelweis seems to have overlooked, confirms Semmelweis's skepticism about the conscientiousness of the chlorine washings as they were practiced in Prague. "Seyfert wanted to provide the clinicians with conclusive proof that the washings were useless and that it was utterly unthinkable that the infection of patients with cadaverous matter would bring about the puerperal condition. One must know that the majority of those who performed examinations came directly from performing autopsies so that it was very easy for such matter to be conveyed. Indeed, in spite of the so-called washings, the frequency and intensity of the disease in the maternity hospital did not diminish. But for me this did not suffice as proof against Dr. Semmelweis's views, for I saw with my own eyes that normally nothing resembling a true washing was involved. As a rule the fingertips were dipped once into a dark liquid that had been used for the same purpose for several days . . . many of the students discontinued even this operation and washed with plain water. Georg Martius, "Mittheilungen aus der Kliniken zu Prag," *Ärztliches Intelligenz-Blatt* 4(1857), 410–15: 410f.

tainly not have been required to wash in chlorine. Perhaps utensils that were used by the diseased were not strictly kept away from the healthy. This could have reduced the effectiveness of the chlorine washings. Finally, decaying matter could have come from the third source. I have explained that, in spite of my caution, at the obstetrical clinic in Pest there were external infections resulting from unclean bed linen. There may also be launderers and attendants in Prague who do not adequately discharge their duties.

[332] Were I in Scanzoni's place and he in mine, I could not say in full honesty that I had seriously practiced chlorine washings. The conclusion that childbed fever does not originate through resorption of decaying matter is, therefore, false. . . .

[333] Scanzoni says further, "We cannot leave it unmentioned that Dr. Semmelweis's hypothesis can have little application in the Prague maternity hospital. Very few mothers are examined after delivery, and moreover, students practicing in the hospital seldom if ever have contact with corpses. This will be confirmed by everyone familiar with the circumstances of the institution."[33] Until now Scanzoni has always spoken of a discovery. His only objection to the facts or inferences on which this discovery is based is that they are not new. Scanzoni nowhere demonstrates that the facts are not true or the inferences erroneous. In his experiments in Prague, Scanzoni found unconfirmed only the last conclusion from these facts and inferences, namely that childbed fever originates through the resorption of decaying matter. His experiments have shown that in March and April of 1848 in the Prague maternity hospital 31 patients died by chance, that in May, with a more favorable *genius epidemicus*, these chance deaths were limited to 1, and that in June, July, and August, 19 patients died without a demonstrable cause. *[334]* For these reasons he now refers to my discovery as an hypothesis. I maintain that I have made a discovery, and believe that the reason why the discovery made in Vienna has been degraded to an hypothesis in Prague is that Scanzoni is not clear about the most important points of this discovery. Of the three sources of decaying

33. Scanzoni, op. cit., note 31 above, pp. 29f.

matter, Scanzoni knows only one; he seems not to be completely clear even about this one, for he says that over the course of many days his students seldom contact corpses. Each student remains two months in the course for practical obstetrics. In Vienna there are 42 students; assume that in Prague there are 20. If only once a week each of these students comes into contact with a corpse, then there are 160 contacts in two months and 960 in a year. If the chlorine washings are poorly done, this number is sufficient to explain not only the acknowledged cases of puerperal fever, but also the 31 patients who died by chance and the 19 who died without a demonstrable cause.

Scanzoni says that this hypothesis also has no application in Prague because very few mothers are examined after delivery. I can assure Scanzoni that in Vienna, too, very few mothers are examined after delivery, but through this remark Scanzoni proves that he is in error about where and when resorption takes place. Resorption occurs at the inner surface of the uterus which, as a result of pregnancy, has lost the mucous membrane. Through injury it can certainly occur elsewhere. Resorption occurs during pregnancy when the inner surface is accessible; during birth this occurs most often in the period of dilation. . . .

[335] Scanzoni writes:

Professor Skoda felt obliged to make the Viennese college of medical professors aware of the importance of Dr. Semmelweis's discovery and to admonish them to name a commission that would fulfill the following charges: First, to construct a table indicating the number of deliveries and deaths from month to month. There should also be a sequential list of assistants and students who had served in the maternity hospital. Assistants and students should be contacted to determine which of them occupied themselves with the examination of corpses. From this information Skoda hoped to determine whether the incidence of disease is related to the participation of the assistants and students in autopsies. [336] Second, to identify street births. Those who deliver on the street are examined only in emergency cases, and if Dr. Semmelweis is correct they should, therefore, have a lower incidence of illness. Third, to collect reports establishing whether there are lower mortality rates in hospitals where infections from corpses cannot

take place. Fourth, to undertake animal experiments. The resolution was adopted by the college of professors by a very large
majority and the commission was immediately named.[34] However, because of a protest by the Professor of Obstetrics, the ministry decided against allowing the commission to act. In consequence of this decision, Professor Skoda recommended that
Semmelweis attempt animal experiments.[35]

This decision of the ministry, together with the denial of my
request for a two-year extension in my period of service, illustrates the difficulties I encountered in attempting to free humanity from the scourge of childbed fever. One cannot easily understand why the Professor of Obstetrics protested; the world would
not have held him responsible for the great mortality. Moreover,
this investigation would have shown that just as he did not bear
this guilt, neither did the staff in the second clinic deserve credit
for the lower mortality. . . .

[337–41] . . . Scanzoni writes:

> Moreover, we are certainly not in agreement with Professor Skoda
> in regarding puerperal fever as identical with pyemia. . . . Pro
> fessor Skoda has neglected to prove statistically that puerperal
> fever can really be characterized as pyemia. As long as this is not
> done, inducing pyemia by injecting deleterious matter into the
> vagina [of an animal] is of no use in identifying the cause of the
> illness of maternity patients. Proving that pyemia can be induced
> in this way, incidentally, did not require Dr. Semmelweis's ex
> periments.[36]

[342] Every case of childbed fever, without a single exception,
is pyemia in the sense that in every case decaying matter is resorbed, the resorbed matter disintegrates the blood, and in some
cases the pyemia is fatal even in this state. More often, however,
exudation follows disintegration of the blood. The true cause of
puerperal fever was discovered from the fact that the pathological remains in Kolletschka were identical with those in the corpses

---

34. See above, chap. 1, footnote 12.
35. Scanzoni, op. cit., note 31 above, p. 30.
36. Ibid., p. 31.

of maternity patients. The cause of Kolletschka's disease was decaying matter; we found the same decaying matter on the hands of the examiners. Kolletschka received the matter from a knife; most patients in maternity hospitals receive it from the examiner. By destroying decaying matter, the disease becomes less frequent. Because of these experiments I no longer regard puerperal fever as a disease that only maternity patients can contract. For me puerperal fever is the same disease that occurs whenever decaying matter is resorbed. Even if puerperal fever is not universally recognized as pyemia in this sense, the opinion is nevertheless gaining strength that pyemia, other than puerperal fever, is caused when resorbed decaying matter disintegrates the blood and thereby causes exudation. . . .

[343] Of course, in Scanzoni's sense of 'pyemia' only a minimal number of cases of puerperal fever are pyemic. I have already shown, however, that Scanzoni provides a defective, entirely worthless classification of puerperal inflammations; for him the essence of childbed fever is *terra incognita*. I can prove statistically that all cases of puerperal fever are pyemia in my sense. Each year from 1841 until 1846 more patients died in Prague than died in the first clinic. The additional deaths, totaling 1,709, were all cases of pyemia in my sense. Even 45 of the deaths in the first clinic in 1848 were cases of pyemia because I was not successful in preventing all cases of external infection. Moreover, in those cases where no decaying matter was introduced externally, decaying matter was generated internally, and so these cases were also pyemia in my sense. Having proved statistically that all cases of childbed fever are cases of pyemia, I repeat my claim that in respect to discovering the cause of the illness of patients, it is extremely valuable to show experimentally that injecting decaying matter into the vagina produces pyemia. . . .

[344] . . . Since Scanzoni has disdained to learn from me, I will evaluate his attempts to dispel the obscurity of puerperal epidemics. [345] For this purpose I communicate Scanzoni's petition to the Bohemian Provincial Government.

Every humane physician desires to know how the frequent and malicious outbreaks of childbed fever in the Imperial Prague Maternity Hospital can be prevented. Humanity has a justified right to expect the government to pursue every apparent solution to this question and to use every means to explore the essence of this horrible yet mysterious disease.

During his more than five years of service in the Prague hospital, your respectful petitioner has become convinced that all the measures that are being or that have been employed to identify the essence of this disease have failed entirely to achieve their purpose. Thus the petitioner, being intimately familiar with the objective manifestations of this disease, and as a member of the examining commission held in the maternity hospital last month, presumes to recommend those measures that appear most suitable for official adoption as leading to determination of the nature of the disease. The adoption of these measures seems all the more pressing, since the Prague hospital, and thereby indirectly the Imperial Provincial Government, has been criticized for being indolent in the face of numerous illnesses and deaths in the maternity hospital, and for making no thorough attempts to shed light on the nature and origin of this malicious disease.

One must first decide with certainty whether the frequent manifestations of puerperal fever are merely epidemic, derived from cosmic and terrestrial conditions, or follow from a miasmatic influence that is dependent on the grouping together of large numbers of maternity patients, or whether the disease is due to a contagium and is spread by infection. It therefore appears to your respectful petitioner that the following measures should be adopted: *[346]* First, before all else, a commission of physicians should be established to examine for at least one year the causes of origin of puerperal fever both inside and outside the hospital. It would be desirable for the members of this commission to be selected by free election from the medical faculty at Prague. In this way the results of their investigations would be regarded as the expression of a learned body of chosen and trusted persons, and so gain credibility and conviction among the medical and lay public. Second, the incidence of sickness and death of women who deliver in the city but outside the hospital should be examined. Thus all the physicians in Prague, both private and officially appointed, should report the requisite information to local officials exactly as is done for other diseases that occur epidemically. Each report should include a brief case history of the sickness and birth with particular attention to the causal factor of the disease.

Third, to answer the question whether the propagation and spread of the disease is due to an infection, experiments should be made on newly delivered female animals (rabbits, dogs, cats, cows). Some of these should be brought into the rooms, indeed into the beds, of patients suffering from puerperal fever, and some should be injected with various secretions from puerperae (lochia, blood, ichor) to test the operation of the harmful matter. *[347]* According to the opinion of your respectful petitioner, only unbiased and open experiments of this kind are persuasive, and it appears that this most obvious measure has not yet been considered by anyone.

Because these proposals can be carried out without any particular difficulties, and because every physician would certainly be pleased to help resolve this important and interesting controversy, the petitioner feels himself pressed with particular urgency, unless theoretical objections can be raised against these measures, to urge their adoption. This is especially the case since if the disease should prove to be contagious, then maternity hospitals would be state-supported deathtraps. However, if puerperal fever proves not to be contagious, as seems more than likely to your respectful petitioner, then the causal operation of cosmic and terrestrial influences will be all the more certainly demonstrated. In this way the Provincial Government would acquit itself of any reproach regarding the correctness of the operation of the maternity hospital. The petitioner is firmly convinced, whatever the results of the examination may be, that the Imperial Provincial Government and the commission of physicians established thereby will provide an immortal service to humanity and to science by solving this important question.[37]

[348] From this petition we see the truth of my claim that the Prague maternity hospital has seen more tragic times than the fifteen months reported by Scanzoni. One would not speak as Scanzoni does of a mortality rate only 1 percent higher than I achieved in Vienna. From the petition we [also] see that Scanzoni's program is not complete. Scanzoni wants to ascertain whether puerperal fever is epidemic, miasmatic, contagious, or infectious. Scanzoni has shown us, through experiments more sagacious than responsible, that in March and April 1848 thirty-

37. Ibid., pp. 31–33. The petition is dated 29 March 1849.

one patients died by chance of puerperal fever, and that in June, July, and August nineteen patients died of puerperal fever without a demonstrable cause. I believe that etiological factors from which thirty-one patients die within two months and nineteen patients die within three months are sufficiently important to be included in a program exploring the causes of childbed fever. The program should, therefore, have been described as follows: finally we will determine when puerperal fever kills by chance, and under what circumstances the causes of childbed fever are absolutely not demonstrable. The petition proves the truth of my claim that Scanzoni is more concerned about who gets credit [*Rechthalberei*] than about discovering the truth. Instead of accepting my discovery that childbed fever always occurs by infection and that every case of childbed fever is a case of resorption fever, he wants to explore the mysteries of childbed fever for himself. For this purpose he proposes to follow the same path that I have followed, even though he has said that he is not in agreement with it.

[349–50] . . . Scanzoni intends to explore the true causes of puerperal fever by commissioning all the physicians in Prague to register with the local government the cause of each case of puerperal fever they encounter. Scanzoni thereby assumes that the physicians know more about the etiology of childbed fever than he knows himself. Except in making a joke, doesn't a person generally ask information from one who knows more than the person doing the asking?[38] In this respect I do not share Scanzoni's opinion. I believe that the physicians in Prague would report what they have learned in school. They would report that so-and-so many became ill and died because of the *genius epidemicus*, that one woman died of puerperal fever because she arose from bed too soon, that another became ill because of a faulty

---

38. Once again Semmelweis is ridiculing a notion that would be unacceptable to us but that seemed perfectly reasonable to Semmelweis's contemporaries. If one believes that the cause of some particular instance of the disease will be some anomaly in the patient's history and that such causes may vary enormously from case to case, then it is not unreasonable to expect physicians to examine individual case histories, report the causes they identify, and then from these reports, determine those causes that are most frequently involved.

diet, that yet another became ill because she received too many visitors, etc. From things that [are generally believed to] have no relation to childbed fever [for example, contamination by decaying organic matter] they will have heard nothing in school, because in school their time was occupied by more wholesome [*heilsameren*] matters. The physicians of Prague would not indicate in their reports that the woman who received too many visitors called her midwife just as the midwife returned from administering douches to a patient with septic endometritis. They would reject as insignificant the fact that the woman with the faulty diet called an obstetrician who, half an hour earlier, had treated a woman with discharging medullary carcinoma of the uterus. They would find it irrelevant that the woman who arose from her bed too early had an obstetrician who, in making the rounds of his other patients, daily cleaned a gangrenous wound, etc. *[351]* I doubt whether Scanzoni would succeed in deriving from the reports of the physicians the true cause of childbed fever. He was not successful in deriving the true cause from Skoda's lecture, which did, of course, refer to things that have no relation to the disease. . . .

[352–55] In summary, Scanzoni's opposition to my theory leaves unchallenged the grounds for rejecting the epidemic theory of childbed fever, and the grounds for adopting my theory. He mentions these grounds and then ignores them. However, the epidemic theory of childbed fever and my grounds for rejecting it cannot both be true. I stand by my beliefs. The theory of epidemic childbed fever is a dangerous error. Since Scanzoni has not proven the contrary, I remain firm in my conviction. . . .

[356] . . . I will now make the counterprobe and determine whether the traditional nonsense, hitherto known as the etiology of childbed fever, which Scanzoni ruminates in both editions of his textbook on obstetrics, can withstand my attack or whether it will collapse like a house of cards.

I first attack the mistake-ridden classification of inflammations among maternity patients; Scanzoni has copied this from earlier writers because the nature of puerperal fever is unknown to him. The success of the chlorine washings proves that inflammation of maternity patients, which Scanzoni does not recognize as puerperal fever, originates through the resorption of decaying matter. Since these cases can be prevented by chlorine washing, they are genuine cases of puerperal fever. The same fact allows us to dispense with [Scanzoni's] entire etiology for these cases. For if these inflammations were grounded in the etiological factors to which Scanzoni ascribes them, then they could not be prevented by chlorine washings. Chlorine washings protect against the resorption of decaying matter but not against the factors that Scanzoni cites. Among other causal factors Scanzoni ascribes these inflammations to the trauma of birth; indeed, he even refers to the infections as traumatic. *[357]* How can the trauma of birth be made harmless by washing one's hands in chlorine? . . .

Scanzoni's theory entails that the trauma of foul decidual or placental remains or blood clots causes a local inflammation that can be converted into regular puerperal fever when the products of the local inflammation are resorbed. Thus, according to Scanzoni, local inflammation occurs first, and may or may not be followed by resorption of the products of the local inflammation. In the former case, the resorbed products may occasion blood disintegration from whence new exudations arise. He says he has observed hundreds of such cases just from endometritis in the Prague hospital. *[358]* However, since we have proven that one can protect against these hundreds of cases, they arise through resorption of decaying matter.

We will now consider the etiology of what Scanzoni recognizes as genuine puerperal fever. Scanzoni says, "Kiwisch claims that the puerperal condition of the woman is the first necessary condition for puerperal fever. However, certainly no one will agree who has had extensive experience and made numerous observations regarding this condition."[39] . . . I agree with Scanzoni when he claims, against Kiwisch, that the puerperal state is not a necessary condition for the origin of puerperal fever. . . . *[359]* As Scanzoni correctly observes, this follows from the fact that puerperal fever can originate and prove fatal during birth, and

39. Wilhelm Friedrich Scanzoni, *Lehrbuch der Geburtshilfe*, 3d ed. (Vienna: L. W. Seidel, 1855), vol. 3, p. 1,004.

even during pregnancy. The first postmortem Caesarean section that I performed was on a woman who died of puerperal fever during pregnancy. But this follows also from the fact that one encounters the disease that I call puerperal fever, namely, the disease that originates from the resorption of deleterious matter, even in individuals who do not have the slightest similarity to the puerperal state. For example, anatomists, surgeons, males and nonpuerperal females who are operated on in surgical wards may contract the disease if they resorb deleterious matter. However, Scanzoni is not correct in saying that the essential predisposing cause of childbed fever is the blood mixture characteristic of pregnancy. If this were so, then puerperal fever could not be prevented by washing the hands in chlorine; chlorine washings do not alter blood mixtures. . . . Moreover, since anatomists, surgeons, and those treated surgically are not puerperae, they do not have the blood mixture characteristic of pregnancy. *[360]* The only characteristic predisposing cause of puerperal fever is a resorbing surface for the resorption of deleterious matter. . . .

[361–63] [Next Semmelweis criticizes Scanzoni's remarks on the etiology of epidemic childbed fever.] Scanzoni observes that it is unfortunate that our investigations of the atmospheric-terrestrial-cosmic factors [supposedly responsible for epidemic fever] have not, as yet, given us much positive understanding of these phenomena. Naturally, one cannot have much positive understanding of that which does not exist. . . . *[364–65]* . . . Scanzoni says the epidemic influence reveals itself not only in the number of those who become ill, but also in the form of the illness. In many epidemics all cases have the character of hyperinosis, in others of pyemia, and in others of disintegration of the blood. Indeed, even the localization reveals epidemic influences, because at different times autopsies reveal lymphangitis, phlebitis, etc. According to Scanzoni, all these circumstances leave no doubt that certain atmospheric influences, whose essences of course are not yet known, are the most significant causal factors of puerperal fever. What Scanzoni says regarding the forms of puerperal fever can be read in many textbooks on obstetrics but cannot be observed in nature. Before 1847 I also had the misfortune of conducting autopsies of many corpses of puerperae. I

gave special attention to the forms in which puerperal fever appeared, because at that time an assistant in the Institute of Pathological Anatomy hoped to form prognoses as to whether the epidemic was beginning, at the acme, or in a state of decline, and whether the epidemic was recidivous, etc. Naturally his prognoses were never fulfilled, and I abandoned all hope for such predictions. But in order to convince myself, over a long period of time, I dissected all the patients who died. *[366]* On days when I had the misfortune of dissecting many corpses I found forms of the beginning, the middle, and the end of the epidemic; there were also forms indicating recidivism. I never found a constant, dominating form during an epidemic. When I finally discovered the true cause of childbed fever, it became entirely conceivable why I was unable to draw conclusions about the effects of a cause that did not, in fact, produce those effects. . . .

[367–69] Scanzoni says this about individuality: "During an epidemic, individual dispositions to disease are less significant; one is not protected by age, constitution, or the circumstances of one's life. Very often the most healthy, youthful, and strong women contract this virulent and fatal disease."[40] The attentive reader knows that puerperal fever epidemics consist of several women being exposed in one way or another to decaying matter. Decaying matter is so horrible a poison that certainly no aspects of the individual can provide protection. Other than during epidemics, Scanzoni believes that the weak, the poorly nourished, those exposed to need and misery during pregnancy, and the emotionally deprived are more susceptible to puerperal fever. I am convinced that none of these circumstances cause the individual either to receive decaying matter from external sources or to generate it internally. These circumstances, therefore, are not etiological factors of childbed fever. How many of the 3,556 patients treated in 1848 in the first clinic satisfied Scanzoni's description? Yet only 45 were lost to puerperal fever. . . .

[370] According to Scanzoni, individuals contract puerperal fever more readily if, during pregnancy, they suffer from a disease that causes a composition of the blood similar to that of one

40. Ibid., p. 1,006.

of the forms of puerperal fever. Women who suffer from pneumonia, pleurisy, pericarditis, or from acute rheumatism [supposedly] belong in this category. If Scanzoni believes that these inflammations bring about a blood composition similar to that of puerperal fever, he is simply proving again that he still does not understand the nature of puerperal fever. Those who die of pyemia, for example anatomists, surgeons, those operated on in surgical wards, or the newborn, have a blood composition identical with that encountered in puerperal fever, but those suffering from the inflammations mentioned by Scanzoni do not. On the contrary, these inflammations protect the patient from puerperal fever. Out of compassion such individuals are not used for instruction, and so they are not infected. Scanzoni also observes that advanced tuberculosis protects one from puerperal fever, because none of the hundreds of puerperal fever victims he has autopsied had advanced tuberculosis. The reason is simply that such patients are not used for instruction, and therefore they are not infected. Scanzoni says that puerperal fever occurs seldom among those suffering from anemia, dropsy, typhoid, scurvy, or acute exanthemata such as smallpox, measles, or scarlet fever. The reason is that such patients are not used for instruction, and therefore they are not infected. If Scanzoni has not observed this from those suffering from the diseases he mentions, then he has not been adequately observant—a fact that would not be surprising. *[371]* Scanzoni has seen many patients die, and from 1847 until 1853 he has had time to reflect and to read much in support of my theory, but all this was not sufficient to enable him to observe that puerperal fever is not epidemic.

All serious diseases protect the patient from puerperal fever in the same way as do street births and premature deliveries. Those who delivered in the street were not used for instruction, since there was nothing to learn from them; those who delivered prematurely were not used for instruction, in hopes that delivery could be delayed. Thus these persons were not infected. . . . This does not mean, however, that ill persons could not contract childbed fever if infection should occur. An exception was eclampsia [coma and (usually) convulsions in pregnant women often associated with hypertension] because eclampsiatics were repeatedly examined in order to determine the correct time to induce birth. Before the adoption of chlorine washings, nearly all eclampsiatics died of childbed fever; thereafter puerperal fever was rare among them.

I agree with Scanzoni that protracted delivery is an etiological factor for childbed fever. I do not agree, however, on how the disease originates in such cases. *[372]* Before all else, one must distinguish whether the period of dilation or the period of labor is extended. If the period of dilation is extended, then the resorbant surface of the uterus remains accessible for a longer period of time; in such cases, the danger of infection from external sources is more serious. . . . During extended labor, infection from external sources cannot occur because the infant makes the resorbant surface of the uterus inaccessible. However, extended labor can cause childbed fever through self-infection; pressure over an extended period can cause partial necrosis; decaying matter may then be produced and resorbed. . . . *[373]* . . . Scanzoni publishes a table of Simpson's showing that mortality of the mother is in direct relation to the length of the birth process. This table would have had more value had it taken into account which part of the birth process is extended. . . .

[374] . . . Emotional disturbances do not cause individuals to receive decaying matter from external sources, and they do not cause its internal generation; thus these are not etiological factors. *[375]* Scanzoni says, "Every active physician is able to cite experiences demonstrating that the health of patients is as seriously threatened by powerfully exciting or depressing emotions as by any other harmful influence."[41] I am an active physician. I observe that women in their first pregnancy, and in subsequent pregnancies as well, are troubled by emotional disturbances— particularly at the end of pregnancy they fear death. However, among the cases for which I am responsible, I observe emotional disturbances so much more frequently than puerperal fever that I cannot reasonably assume that there is any connection between them. . . . Scanzoni also says:

> Supported by repeated experiences, I myself fear nothing so much as when a patient is suddenly seized by great fear, anger, or worry. For there is, perhaps, no phase of life in which such emotions are

41. Ibid., p. 1,007.

more harmful than immediately after birth. *[376]* I have observed
many cases in which there is no doubt that such an emotional
disturbance provided the essential cause of puerperal sickness. This
ordinarily goes as follows: immediately after the operation of this
harmful influence, a violent chill occurs, the physiognomy becomes characteristically distorted, and with a sudden loss of
strength all the manifestations of a rapidly developing disintegration of the blood appear. These emotional disturbances are particularly to be feared when they befall a patient who is already ill;
then, more than at any other time, is the onset of a lethal disintegration of the blood to be feared.[42]

Scanzoni has so often shown himself to be such a wretched observer that I cannot accept his observation regarding the connection between emotional disturbance and puerperal fever. I am
much more of the opinion that in his many observed cases, either
he or someone else infected the patient and that between the time
of the infection and the outbreak of fever, emotional disturbances occurred. . . .

[377–93] . . . At the conclusion of his treatment of the etiology of childbed fever Scanzoni writes:

> I hold the influence, which so often encloses the maternity hos-
> pitals in its murderous power, to be miasmatic. However, I must
> add that atmospheric, in other words epidemic, influences cannot
> be denied. In support of this I must mention that frequent sick-
> nesses in the hospital often coincide with puerperal epidemics
> outside; both increase and decline together. And it frequently
> happens that with a sudden change in the weather or other at-
> mospheric alterations, the disease stops, even in institutions where
> for some time it has remained constant.[43]

The murderous influence in maternity hospitals is not found in
puerperal miasma but in decaying matter. Not to mention the
experiences of others, this is proven by my having ended the
murderous influence at three institutions by measures directed
not against puerperal miasma but against decaying matter. If

42. Ibid.
43. Ibid., p. 1,010.

Scanzoni identifies the murderous influence as puerperal miasma, he incriminates himself and all directors whose maternity institutions are subject to this murderous influence. For it would have been their most holy duty to prevent the development of this miasma or, once it had come into existence, to destroy it. *[394]* The maternity hospitals are state-supported deathtraps, not only if puerperal fever is contagious but also if it is miasmatic or infectious. I am of the conviction that puerperal fever never originates other than by infection. Because of this conviction, since 1847 I have done everything in my power to prevent maternity hospitals from being deathtraps. Scanzoni believes that puerperal miasma is the murderous influence in the maternity hospitals, and nevertheless, he utters not a syllable as to how one can prevent or destroy the miasma. This reflects Scanzoni's thoughtlessness in writing about things he does not understand. . . .

[395] . . . Scanzoni indicates that puerperal fever is not a contagious disease; I agree. Scanzoni writes:

> All the evidence cited in favor of the contagiousness of puerperal fever is either unproven, or is compatible with the idea that deleterious matter from a diseased patient causes a general morbid condition of the blood of healthy patients. . . . This last-named method of generation of puerperal fever has recently been brought to the attention of the medical public by Semmelweis and Skoda. They claim that the unfavorable health at the first obstetrical clinic in Vienna was due only to the condition that shortly before examining patients, physicians had been engaged in the morgue, and that they conveyed deleterious particles adhering to their hands onto the genitals of those they examined. *[396]* I was the first to contest this opinion. Shortly thereafter I was joined, at least in the essential points, by [Bernhard] Seyfert, Kiwisch, [Eduard] Lumpe, and Zipfl. Also the discoveries that Arneth published in Paris in the proceedings of the Academy did not support Semmelweis. . . . I do not contest the possibility that isolated infections can occur in this way, but one goes too far in maintaining that the frequency and virulence of puerperal sickness in the maternity institutions can be explained entirely in this way.[44] . . .

44. Ibid.

[397] . . . Scanzoni says Lumpe and Zipfl have agreed with him. The facts are these. On 15 May 1850, at the general meeting of the Imperial Society of Physicians in Vienna, I delivered a lecture on the origin and prevention of childbed fever. A discussion followed that was continued at the general meeting on 18 June and concluded at the general meeting on 15 July.[45] *[398]* In this discussion Lumpe and Zipfl spoke against me. But Chiari, Arneth, Helm, and [Anton] Hayne supported my position, and Dr. [Heinrich] Herzfelder, the first secretary of the society, wrote the following in his report of the meeting:

> In general pathology we encounter what appears to be the practical solution to one of the greatest responsibilities of medicine, namely Dr. Semmelweis's discovery of the cause of the origin of the previously devastating puerperal epidemics. According to his opinion, childbed fever originates only through the resorption of foul organic matter into the blood of the mother, and this matter, unless it is generated internally, comes from external sources. Most often it comes from the dissection of corpses and is transmitted to the female organs by the obstetricians themselves. For this reason Semmelweis has ordered thorough washings with chlorine solution before every delivery. In this way he has been fortunate enough to halt the spread of the previously serious epidemic. Doctors Zipfl and Lumpe provided powerful and praiseworthy opposition to this view of the origin of the disease; they sought to vindicate the miasmatic origin of this evil by the use of statistical data. In the discussion, however, this view, as that of Scanzoni and Seyfert of Prague, was sufficiently refuted. Thus, this conception of the disease, most warmly defended by Doctors Arneth, Chiari, Helm, and, from the point of view of animal medicine, by Professor Hayne, can be recognized as a true triumph of medical discovery.[46] . . .

45. The text of Semmelweis's lecture was not published, but there were minutes of the lecture and of the following discussions. *Zeitschrift der k. k. Gesellschaft der Ärzte zu Wien* 6, no. 2(1850): cxxxvii–cxl, clxvi–clxix; 7, no. 1(1851):iii–x. These are reprinted in Györy, op. cit., note 4 above, pp. 49–58.

46. Heinrich Herzfelder, "Bericht über die Leistungen der k. k. Gesellschaft der Ärzte in Wien während des Jahres 1850," [*Zeitschrift der k. k. Gesellschaft der Ärzte zu Wien* 8(1851): vii; author's note].

[399–400] . . . The reader has seen how poorly Scanzoni's etiology withstands criticism. With the exception of a few facts that Scanzoni has correctly observed, and with the exception of a few isolated cases where Scanzoni will not deny infection, all the rest appears to be a mass of error and confusion. It would have been good fortune indeed for the birthgiving sex if there were no etiology of childbed fever except that which Scanzoni recognizes. For certainly no patient has ever died of childbed fever as a result of epidemic influences, and no patient has ever died as a result of her individuality. Mothers and infants have died of childbed fever as a result of protracted labor, but certainly not as Scanzoni imagines it. . . . No patients have died of childbed fever as a result of emotional disturbances, of mistakes in diet, or of a puerperal miasma, because puerperal miasma does not exist as Scanzoni conceives it. *[401]* What then was the etiological factor from which so many hundreds died at the Prague hospital? The reader will recall that in Scanzoni's sagacious and conscientious experiments with chlorine washings, two important etiological factors were discovered; namely, it was communicated that in March and April of 1848, thirty-one patients died by chance, and in June, July, and August of 1848, nineteen patients died without a demonstrable cause. If, therefore, these many hundreds of patients whose autopsies Scanzoni attended died partly by chance and partly without any demonstrable cause, and if my criticisms of Scanzoni's etiology are erroneous, then Scanzoni himself is at fault. For in his secrecy he has not taught me and the rest of the world about these two causal factors that he has discovered and that are so important in his etiology.

[402] In 1847 I discovered that puerperal fever originates through infection. In 1850 Scanzoni described my discovery as an hypothesis. In 1852, in the first edition of his textbook on obstetrics, Scanzoni explained that he did not contest the possibility that isolated cases could occur through this kind of infection. In the second edition of his textbook, which appeared in 1853, he remained of the same opinion. In 1854 the fourth edition of Kiwisch's *Clinical Lectures* appeared, edited and expanded by Scanzoni. Kiwisch says the following about the prophylaxis

of childbed fever: "As conscientiously as possible, one should prevent infecting maternity patients in any way with decaying animal matter (poison from corpses, secretions from wounds, decaying maternity effluvium). For this purpose one may recommend chlorine washings and fumigation, practices that have been adopted by the English and by Dr. Semmelweis."[47] Although this statement of Kiwisch's refers only to cases of infection from external causes, although he ignores all cases of self-infection, and although chlorine washings and fumigation cannot prevent all cases of infection from external causes, nevertheless Kiwisch's statement surpasses Scanzoni's opinion that only isolated cases of infection are not to be contested. Scanzoni does not contradict this statement in his editorial comments, as he does some of Kiwisch's other statements; I take this as a favorable sign that Scanzoni is being converted to my opinion. . . .

[403] . . . Toward the end of 1859 an essay by Dr. H. Silberschmidt appeared under the title *Critical Historical Representation of the Pathology of Childbed Fever.* The author of this essay attacks my views on the origin of childbed fever. This essay was awarded a prize by the medical faculty of Würzburg, an association of which Scanzoni is a member; he certainly exerted a decisive influence in this matter. . . . Silberschmidt says, "Skoda and Semmelweis believe the primary cause of childbed fever is poison from corpses."[48] This first sentence proves that Dr. Silberschmidt passes judgment on my opinions without understanding them. The immediate cause of puerperal fever is decaying animal-organic matter. One of the three sources from which this matter is drawn is certainly corpses, and the decaying matter at the first clinic in Vienna was, in fact, taken from corpses more frequently than from the two other sources. . . . [404] In the maternity ward at St. Rochus Hospital the great mortality of

47. Franz Kiwisch von Rotterau, *Klinische Vorträge über specielle Pathologie und Therapie der Krankheiten des weiblichen Geschlectes,* 4th ed. ([Prague: J. G. Calve], 1854), [vol. 1, p. 634; author's note].

48. H. Silberschmidt, *Historisch-kritische Darstellung der Pathologie des Kindbettfiebers von den ältesten Zeiten bis auf die unserige,* ([Erlangen: Ferdinand Enke], 1859), [pp. 177f.; author's note].

maternity patients is explained by the fact that the head surgeon was simultaneously the head obstetrician. The mortality rate in this hospital was dependent on decaying matter generated by the sick. . . . For two years the excessive mortality rate at the Pest obstetrical clinic was caused by decaying matter from the third source. While Chiari directed the Prague maternity hospital, the decaying matter for two epidemics came from two patients whose genitals became gangrenous because of mistreatment during delivery. The decaying matter that caused the first epidemic recognized as such in the history of puerperal fever came from the wounded. Neither Professor Skoda nor I believe that this is the case; on the contrary, we know it to be true. Professor Skoda and I share this conviction, and if Dr. Silberschmidt is capable of conviction, if he does not simply write at the orders of whoever will praise his work, then I recommend to him a fundamental study of this essay. I am certain that he will come to the same conviction.

[405–7] . . . In concluding his efforts in exploring the pathology of puerperal fever through many centuries, Dr. Silberschmidt proclaims as most perfect Scanzoni's hyperinosis, pyemia, and blood dissolution of maternity patients. The reader will recall that in the course of judging Scanzoni I proved statistically (in spite of Scanzoni's claims to the contrary) that inflammation during maternity is genuine puerperal fever, as is hyperinosis, pyemia, and blood dissolution. All of these originate by the resorption of decaying matter. [408] Scanzoni divides these inflammations, which are [supposedly] not puerperal fever, into numerous forms, one of which, namely endometritis, he claims to have observed in hundreds of cases. If, therefore, hundreds of cases of puerperal fever do not belong to Scanzoni's pathology of puerperal fever, the reader has some conception of the perfection of Scanzoni's pathology. . . .

[Semmelweis calculates that his discovery could save thousands of lives; he then addresses Scanzoni directly.] [409] . . . You know, councilor, that I must praise myself because I am not praised by my opponents. In my self-praise, I go so far as to claim that with the exception of Jenner's cowpox inoculations, there is no third discovery in the whole history of medicine that, by protecting against a disease, can save as many human lives as my teaching regarding protection against childbed fever. . . . Then, at the end of 1859, an association—in which you, councilor, certainly exercise a decisive influence—awards a prize to an essay in which the eternal truths I have discovered are attacked so stupidly. . . .

[410] Joseph Steiner, a candidate in surgery and my student in the lectures in theoretical obstetrics, wrote the following to me in Pest:

> Thoroughly convinced of the truth of your lectures on puerperal fever which I had the good fortune to attend in the Winter Semester, I feel it necessary to communicate some speculations as to how infections may be spread at the Graz maternity hospital.
>
> As I attended the first year lectures in surgery at Graz, there was an inn in the general hospital that saw to the needs of the sick. It was also a gathering place for students. Later, however, the Sisters of Charity took over direction of the kitchen and the inn was closed. The students were then obliged to select the dissection room for their gatherings. This room became the place where colleagues met and spent time together before attending lectures. In the afternoons first-year students were obliged to dissect. Students in the other classes, who were required by the regulations to prepare for their oral examinations, frequently came, too, in order to show the beginners how to do their work. . . . Those connected with the maternity ward visited the dissection room most frequently because the maternity ward was separated from the hospital only by a street. One could not criticize those who made examinations in the maternity ward if, instead of remaining there twenty-four hours at a time, they came into the dissecting room for diversion. It often happened that a poor student who was on call and who could not remain away from the maternity ward for long came into the dissecting room to try to get some money for a snack, and then went back to the ward to conduct his rounds. *[411]* The money would be earned by helping a student complete his dissections. It often happened that my brother, who was studying practical obstetrics, visited me in the dissecting room in order to study the anatomy of corpses with me or to help me conduct a dissection. I had to finish my dissection by a certain time, and he would then return to his rounds in

the maternity ward. I remember one time going back to the maternity ward with my brother. He put down his hat and cane and proceeded to examine a patient. I asked him why he previously spread grease on his hand and he answered that it was to make his hand slippery. I am convinced that I would have noticed had my brother washed his hands with any liquid (as, for example, chloride of lime) because I would have been curious enough to ask what it was. But since I did not ask, my brother must have neglected to wash his hands. This negligence was due to a total ignorance of the origin of puerperal fever; all the advanced students at Graz shared this negligence because they were inclined to look for a completely different kind of cause. Thus such frequent visitors to the dissection room are extremely dangerous to maternity patients. They establish such a communication between the dissecting room and the maternity ward—indeed, I am inclined to say between the dissecting room and the genitals of the patients—as can only exist between two rooms that share a common door. Actually, the patients would have been in less danger in the dissecting room than in the maternity ward. A student would certainly not have examined patients with hands that had just sorted through wet, bloody muscle tissue, he would certainly first clean his hands. Unfortunately, however, the patients are in the maternity ward rather than in the dissecting room. Thus the student must leave the dissecting room in order to carry out the examination. His hands dry in the air or they become dry when he puts them in his pockets a few times, and by the time he arrives in the maternity ward he examines with as much negligence as my brother. *[412]* To me it is no longer a riddle why at one examination the city physician exclaimed that the maternity hospitals are truly institutions of death. I asked a school servant what could have been meant by such a remark. He answered, as though it were the most trivial affair in the world, "Oh well, right now there are a couple more in there on a slab, like fish." Here I have given only conjectures, but from these it seems clear that puerperal fever is a consequence of resorption.[49] . . .

[413–17] . . . We return now to Prague and in particular to Josef Hamernik, a member of the commission to which, in 1849,

49. Graz, 30 March 1858 [author's note].

Scanzoni gave the responsibility of exploring this puzzling disease. How thoroughly this commission explores is easy to surmise from the fact that in 1860 the solution to this puzzle has not yet been revealed to the world; we infer that the exploration is still not complete.

[418] After complaining that our knowledge of etiology is so imperfect, Hamernik says the following: "In order for any purported cause to be recognized as the actual cause of a disease, we must always be able to answer the following questions affirmatively: does this cause always have the same effect? As an experiment can one always bring about the disease in this way? In those cases in which the cause does not bring about the specified disease, can the same reason for failure always be identified?" [50] We will now see whether my etiology of childbed fever satisfies Hamernik's conditions. The first condition is unfounded. The reader knows that I have injected rabbits with decaying matter; some consequently died from pyemia and others did not. Could we deny that the decaying matter was the cause of pyemia in the rabbits that died, simply because the matter did not occasion pyemia in all the rabbits? I have fulfilled the second condition: I have produced puerperal fever experimentally in rabbits in this way. I have not fulfilled the third condition; I cannot explain why a few rabbits did not develop pyemia. However, instead, my etiology of childbed fever satisfies another condition that Hamernik has not posed but one that constitutes a condition for a true etiology. Namely, I have reduced the disease by making harmless that which I have identified as its cause.

Although my etiology achieves more than Hamernik requires, he says the following: "It is entirely fallacious and arbitrary to declare that childbed fever is generated when examiners convey cadaverous particles to maternity patients. *[419]* For childbed fever epidemics are a much older part of medicine than the autopsies of corpses. . . . This was always the horror of mothers, even at times and in countries where no one so much

50. Joseph Hamernik, *Die Cholera epidemica*, (Prague: [Calve], 1850), 247f. [author's note].

as thought about performing post-mortems on corpses."[51] It is really to be regretted that Hamernik, who reveals such a great talent for medical history, has done nothing to develop this special talent. *[420]* For the time being I stand by my conviction that at times and in countries where the etiology I have identified does not yet operate, childbed fever occurs only in isolated cases. . . .

[421–22] . . . In the eighteenth of his *Chemical Letters*, [Justus] Liebig[52] says that

> corpses in anatomical theaters frequently enter a state of decomposition that is then communicated to the blood of a living body. The smallest wound from a knife that has been used in dissection results in a condition that often threatens life (cases are not rare in which persons have been sacrificed to this horrible poison— Dr. Kolletschka in Vienna, Dr. Bender in Frankfurt am Main). [François] Magendie[53] observed that decomposing blood, brain matter, gall, ichor, etc., when applied to a fresh wound, occasion vomiting, weakness, and sooner or later death. This observation has never been contradicted.[54]

In the third appendix to this passage, after a brief excerpt from Skoda's lecture before the Imperial Academy of Vienna, Liebig says, "From this lecture it appears, incidentally, how little attention has been given to this large and practical discovery outside the Academy. Certainly other causes of childbed fever will be identified. However, no unprejudiced person can doubt that the one identified so insightfully by Dr. Semmelweis at the maternity hospital in Vienna is among these causes."[55] *[423]* The uni-

51. Ibid., p. 265.
52. Justus Liebig (1803–73) was a widely known chemist and one of the founders of physiological and agricultural chemistry.
53. François Magendie (1783–1855) was a French physician and the founder of experimental physiology. He distinguished motor and sensory nerves and made important contributions to understanding the operation of the veins.
54. Justus Liebig, *Chemische Briefe*, [(Heidelberg: C. F. Winke, 1851)], p. 312 [author's note].
55. Ibid., p. 714.

versal cause of childbed fever is decaying matter. There are three sources of decaying matter; one of these is corpses. Liebig deleted this passage, so favorable to me, from the second edition of *Chemical Letters*, and I presumed to write asking why. With some trepidation that I might receive an answer expressing surprise at my naivete, I also took the opportunity to ask Liebig for his opinion regarding the disinfective power of chlorine.[56] I became indebted to Liebig for the following reply:

> I am honored to reply to your letter that the omission of your observations regarding childbed fever from the new edition of my *Chemical Letters* was made not because I no longer recognize the importance of your experience. Rather it was because it is now so well and widely known that its retention in my book appeared to have no purpose; it did not relate directly to the subject matter. Other supplementary items have also been left out. There is no doubt that chlorine possesses disinfective qualities.[57] . . .

[424–28] While I was a student of practical obstetrics at the first clinic in Vienna, Chiari was the assistant. In his lectures on puerperal fever he said that epidemic influences were sometimes so intense that even non-puerperae contracted the disease. As proof he cited the case of a person suffering from a fibrous polyp of the uterus who was admitted to the clinic and who died before the operation. Autopsy disclosed the pathological remains of childbed fever. After the consequences of chlorine washings demonstrated how puerperal fever arises, Chiari himself called my attention again to this case with the observation that he now knew that this individual, just like the maternity patients, was infected by decaying matter. The miserable condition of those cared for in gynecological wards is clearly revealed in their operation reports. Individuals with polyp of the uterus often die of pyemia before the operation or after excision. I have directed a

56. Some of Semmelweis's critics questioned the effectiveness of chlorine as a disinfectant. See above, p. 189; German edition, p. 311; and below, p. 239; German edition, p. 494.

57. Munich, 21 March 1859 [author's note].

gynecological institution for six years. In the five years I have been a professor I have myself accepted all those who seek admission with a polyp of the uterus, and in private practice I often have the opportunity to operate on such cases. With one exception I have excised all the numerous polyps; I do not have a single death to report. I have not seen a serious illness after excision, although some [excised polyps] have been as long as the palm of the hand. I attribute this success to the circumstance that I operate only with clean hands. . . .

[429] . . . Kiwisch discussed Skoda's lecture in the Academy of Science at Vienna. He disagreed with Skoda's view that this was a new discovery.

> For many years and from all sides it has been urged that puerperal fever derived from an infection of decaying animal matter and, in particular, from the poison of corpses. This view has been vigorously defended, and would certainly already have been accepted if the physicians who espouse this view had presented conclusive arguments. Thus Dr. Semmelweis sought only to prove that in the Viennese maternity hospital the cause of the frequent disease was primarily deleterious animal matter that was conveyed to the patients. No one can deny that he worked with great patience and achieved considerable success.[58]

[430] It is certainly correct that the English preceded me in observing that decaying matter causes puerperal fever. The limited understanding of English physicians and the substantial difference between their opinions and my own have already been discussed. However, it is abundantly clear that Kiwisch does not even recognize the limited truth known to the English. In his contributions as reviewer for the *Canstattischen Jahresbericht* for 1842 through 1845, Kiwisch reported the observations of the English physicians. . . . In 1845 he made the following comments:

58. Franz Kiwisch von Rotterau, ["Einige Worte über die vom Professor Skoda veröffentlichte Entdeckung des Dr. Semmelweis die Entstehung des Puerperalfiebers betreffend"], *Zeitschrift der k. k. Gesellschaft der Ärzte zu Wien* 6(1850), [300–306]: 300 [author's note].

It must occur to everyone that the observations so frequently communicated by the English doctors are seldom confirmed on the continent; some of the most experienced physicians make no such observations at all. *[431]* Thus, in spite of the rich opportunity afforded by many years of careful study, the reviewer has never been able to collect experiences that would halfway support these observations. After leaving autopsies of persons who died from septic puerperal fever and frequently going directly to examinations of maternity patients, it has never been conclusively demonstrated that this provided any particular disadvantage for patients. The reviewer could never trace the cause of puerperal fever to infection from gangrenous erysipelas. Similarly, in the maternity hospital in which he has worked, it has never been possible to show with probability that anyone ever contracted puerperal fever from a diseased non-maternity patient. The more precise significance of this divergence in experience and opinion must be determined in the future.[59] . . .

The highest mortality rate for the first clinic was 15 percent. Kiwisch regards it as a great service that I reduced this rate. In Würzburg he had a mortality rate of 26 percent and he says, nevertheless, that no disadvantages were observed when he frequently went directly from the autopsy of a victim of septic puerperal fever to examine patients. *[432]* The 26 percent mortality shows that his behavior did not lack disadvantages; only the ability to recognize them was lacking. Kiwisch has no idea of the wholesome truth that lies in the observations of English physicians. . . .

Kiwisch says I performed a great service in reducing the mortality rate of the first clinic. In the same essay he says that he himself pays no attention to whether or not his students come directly from the morgue. Even if Kiwisch had not admitted this it would have been obvious—a mortality rate of 26 percent is possible only in a hospital in which no one pays attention to whether the examiners come directly from the morgue. Kiwisch is blind to the observations of the English. This follows from

59. Franz Kiwisch von Rotterau, *Canstattischen Jahresbericht* [*über die Fortschritte in der Heilkunde im Jahre 1845*, vol. 3, *Specielle Pathologie und Therapie*, (Erlangen: Ferdinand Enke, 1846), pp. 430f.; author's note].

the 1854 edition of his *Clinical Lectures* in which childbed fever is defined as a miasmatic disease.[60] But he is unclear about the import of his own teachings, for he has forgotten to explain how one can prevent the miasma from forming or, when once generated, how it can be destroyed. *[433]* Kiwisch did not know that one can prevent a miasmatic disease. . . .

[434–36] . . . Hermann Lebert is too insignificant an opponent to warrant consideration, but he proves that Kiwisch is wrong in claiming to have known in 1842 what I discovered in 1847. In 1859 Lebert, who was Kiwisch's student, still didn't know how puerperal fever came about. In 1859 Lebert defined childbed fever as follows: "Puerperal fever is a feverish disease characteristic of maternity patients which has a miasmatic origin. It is ultimately a blood disorder which, depending on its various characteristics, occasions a variety of local phenomena (mostly inflamed). In spite of differences, these phenomena generally have the other common characteristic of being localized in the birth organs and then, usually later, in every tissue of the body that is connected with or anatomically similar to the uterus."[61] Regarding that which Kiwisch is supposed to have known in 1842, that is, regarding my teachings, Lebert says the following: "It is questionable whether those who have died of this disease can have been directly inoculated by poison from corpses. Semmelweis has elevated this possibility into a[n entire medical] system. In any case this would be only one of many possibilities of conveyance."[62] . . .

[437–38] In the general meeting of the Imperial Society of Physicians held on 15 May 1850, I presented a lecture on my opinions. The lecture generated a discussion that continued in general meetings on 18 June and 15 July.[63] Dr. Zipfl participated in these discussions as an opponent of my views.

60. Kiwisch, op. cit., note 47 above, 1:600–605.
61. Hermann Lebert, *Handbuch der Praktischen Medicin*, (Tübingen: H. Laupp, 1859), vol. 2, p. 755.
62. Ibid., pp. 759f.
63. See above, note 45.

Dr. Zipfl was assistant in the years 1842 and 1843 in the clinic for midwives. At that time I was an aspirant for assistant in the clinic for physicians, and each morning I made gynecological studies on the female corpses in the morgue. I very frequently saw Dr. Zipfl performing autopsies on the patients who died in the clinic for midwives. I later met Dr. Zipfl at a time when the success of the chlorine washing was known. He congratulated me and assured me that he also had been confused by the disease, that he was confused because things were less clear in the second clinic, and that had he been in the clinic for physicians, where the facts were so convincing, he would certainly have reached the same conclusions. Assured by such expressions, I remarked that the autopsies I had seen him perform had caused the mortality rate in his clinic to reach new highs. *[439]* At the same time I appealed to his love for truth to allow me to use this fact together with his name. Dr. Zipfl willingly agreed and remarked that it was no dishonor to revere pathological anatomy.

I was more than a little surprised when, after I had obtained permission to cite him, Dr. Zipfl participated [in the discussion] as my opponent. He also objected to my suggestion that he had caused such a great mortality. To prove that the autopsies he conducted were not the cause of puerperal fever, Dr. Zipfl collected the reports of autopsies conducted in 1842 on which his name appeared. There were forty-one. He then compared these with birth reports and found that only a few deaths were recorded among those who delivered on days when he performed autopsies, that the fewest became ill from those who delivered a short time after his recorded autopsies, whereas the largest number became ill from those who delivered a longer time (twenty-four to thirty-six hours) after his recorded autopsies.

I have seen Dr. Zipfl performing autopsies so frequently that I am convinced that of the 202 patients who died in the midwives clinic during 1842, only a few were not dissected. If only forty-one autopsies were reported, this merely shows that because the remains were similar, most of the autopsies were not recorded. On days when no autopsies were recorded, patients were infected from unrecorded autopsies. Moreover, in saying that individuals who delivered later became ill and died, Zipfl confirms my theory; those who delivered immediately after the autopsies were in the process of delivery when they were examined and were protected from infection by the inaccessibility of the inner surface of the uterus. Those who delivered later were examined during dilation and, because of the accessibility of the inner surface of the uterus, they became infected. . . .

[440–43] . . . Dr. Lumpe writes,

When one thinks how, since the first occurrence of puerperal fever epidemics, observers of all times have sought in vain for its causes and the means of preventing it, Semmelweis's theory takes on the appearance of the egg of Columbus.[64] I myself was originally overjoyed as I heard the fortunate results of the chlorine washings; as everyone else, I, too, have had the misfortune to witness many blossoming young women fall before this devastating plague. However, during my two years as assistant in the first clinic, I observed incredible variations in the incidence of sickness and death. Because of this I had many doubts about this theory of the origin and prophylaxis of the disease. The more sharply I focused my attention on these doubts, the more clearly they stood forth as logical contradictions. In the face of these doubts, the pious hopes of humanity do not justify accepting theories [like Semmelweis's] as exact science.[65]

I am entirely of Dr. Lumpe's opinion when he says that my theory is like the egg of Columbus. I myself have often expressed amazement, not at my having become aware of the strident contradiction between theory and daily observation, but rather that it was not recognized long before me. . . .

64. At one point Columbus challenged a group of courtiers to stand an egg on end. After they tried without success, Columbus siezed the egg and mashed its end onto the table; the egg, of course, remained upright. The story epitomizes success achieved by transcending the limitations that are assumed to accompany a given problem. Lumpe's point is that Semmelweis has trivially solved the problem of childbed fever by recharacterizing the disease and by adopting a measure that would eliminate all those cases that satisfy the new characterization (but, perhaps, fail completely to prevent the cases that were included under the original characterization of the disease).

65. [Eduard] Lumpe, ["Zur Theorie der Puerperalfieber"], *Zeitschrift der k. k. Gesellschaft der Ärzte zu Wien* 6 [1850, 392–98]: 392 [author's note].

[444–45] . . . Dr. Lumpe says, "Let us see how the facts line up with the unremitting demands of logic." Lumpe says that during his service there were such vast differences between the maximum and minimum mortality rates "that any other possibility is more plausible than one common and constant cause."[66] The common cause of all cases of puerperal fever that ever have been or ever will be is certainly decaying animal-organic matter. However, if Dr. Lumpe claims that recognizing a common cause means that those occupied in the maternity hospital are always contaminated to the same degree, and that consequently the mortality should not fluctuate, then this is a claim that bears all the characteristics of trashy [*Lumpe'schen*[67]] exact science. . . .

[446–50] . . . "With theories of puerperal fever," says Lumpe, "it is as it is with all theories. For example, physicists once explained light by the theory of emanations; now it is explained by the theory of vibrations. Who guarantees that this is right?"[68] Light behaves as it must, undaunted by the explanations of physicists. But puerperal fever is very much dependent on the theories of physicians. Dr. Lumpe explains the origin of puerperal fever by epidemic influences and he sends nearly one patient to the morgue each day. I explain the origin of puerperal fever by infection with decaying matter and in 1848 I sent only forty-five patients to the morgue. Among these were at least ten who could have been saved had I not been obliged to work under inclement circumstances. If I were concerned only with giving yet another explanation for a mortality rate that remains unaffected thereby, then I would find better uses for my time than contending with the errors and ill will of my opponents.

Dr. Lumpe says, "Semmelweis believes that the higher mortality rate in the first clinic conclusively proves his view. Semmelweis ignores one obvious circumstance that seems to me to be of the highest importance: patients were admitted to the first clinic four days a week, two of these days being successive, while they were admitted to the second only three days. Thus, it was

66. Ibid., p. 393.
67. *Lumpen* in German means rags or trash. Semmelweis is punning on Lumpe's name.
68. Ibid., p. 396.

virtually impossible for the rooms in the first clinic to be thoroughly aired out, while this occurred regularly in the second."[69] *[451]* I have not discussed this circumstance because it has no relation to the mortality rate in the first clinic. Only a science as exact as Lumpe's can assign this circumstance such a high importance. If Lumpe is really convinced that because of this circumstance he sent nearly one patient a day to the morgue, then how will he explain his criminal neglect in not so much as proposing that such an easy expedient be attempted. . . .

[452–53] . . . After Lumpe has proved that mortality varies inversely with the opportunity to contaminate the hands, after he has proved that patients who are most frequently examined are least likely to die, he concludes that he has reduced my teachings to absurdity and that he will maintain, throughout all eternity, that contaminated fingers cannot explain infection. After he has proved all this so convincingly, Lumpe says,

> Because of everything that has been said, I deny that infection from corpses is the single and true cause of puerperal fever; nevertheless, I still do not regard chlorine washings as superfluous. *[454]* If adoption of the washings makes it possible to avoid even the least significant of the many concurring factors that cause puerperal fever, then their initial adoption was a sufficiently large service. However, whether this is in fact the case, only the future will be able to decide. In the meantime, I believe we should wait and wash.[70] . . .

[455–59] . . . Joseph Hermann Schmidt, Professor of Obstetrics in Berlin, wrote the following in an editorial:

> A normal birth is often a slow process, and it would be unreasonable to expect every young man involved in the process to remain in the delivery room from the first labor pain until the final conclusion of the birth process. In this respect, therefore, it is very convenient that maternity wards are under the same roof as other clinics. *[460]* Students of obstetrics are thus able to go alternatively into medical or surgical wards or into special clinics and

69. Ibid.
70. Ibid., pp. 397f.

occasionally return to determine what progress has been made. Or they can also go into the morgue from whence they can be quickly called if significant changes occur. . . .

In this regard I received the following letter from my dear friend and colleague, Professor Brücke in Vienna. . . . "In the Viennese maternity hospital many patients have died over the years from puerperal fever. In particular they have died in the clinic for male students, while the mortality in the clinic for midwives is small. This large mortality has occasioned Dr. Semmelweis to forbid any student from examining patients during or after delivery unless that student first washes with a solution of chlorine and soda. He believes that puerperal fever often arises when students manually examine patients after having participated in dissections of corpses and without having thoroughly cleaned their hands. In fact it is striking that the large mortality has occurred here since pathological anatomy has been diligently pursued, and that pathological anatomy has not been studied in the second clinic. *[461]* The Academy of Science has commissioned me to investigate. In the interests of science and humanity I therefore write to ask you whether in your institution or in that directed by Professor [Dietrich Wilhelm Heinrich] Busch there have been experiences that would support the opinion expressed by Dr. Semmelweis." To my regret I could communicate to Herr Brücke no more than my belief that such is possible. . . .

[462] At first glance one could say that the Westphalian farm woman seen in private practice has an advantage over the woman in a Berlin hospital; the cadaverous miasma has never come into her living vagina, while here the fingers of the examining students bring this directly from the morgue. *[463]* But on more careful consideration this hypothesis poses the following simple question: of the many normal deliveries, why do so relatively few suffer from septic metritis, etc., given that they are so frequently examined by students? Thus I believe, nevertheless, that the nosocomial atmosphere[71] of the maternity wards, and not the cadavers of the morgue, must be the object of criticism when, after carelessness, metritis or peritonitis occur. We also segregate

71. "Nosocomial" means originating or taking place in a hospital. A nosocomial atmosphere was a particularly harmful atmospheric influence believed to originate in hospitals and because of which patients who were relatively healthy when admitted could become ill.

midwives from obstetricians, but they were first separated in 1846. We have not carefully determined the difference in mortality rates between the two divisions; Semmelweis initiated this approach. He conducted experiments on rabbits; one may not conduct such experiments on people. Thus direct counter evidence is impossible. In response to this hypothetical etiology, Semmelweis himself employed the apparently reliable prophylaxis of chlorinated soda. Before touching the internal organs of the living, everyone must disinfect himself with this solution if he has worked with corpses. In the future this inexpensive requirement will be adopted into practice by every obstetrical clinic, and the opportunity to do this will be provided by individual washing stands.

As mentioned, I believe in the possibility, and for me the Viennese experience is totally sufficient to warrant caution. I do not demand details. It may be that this is one path that leads to childbed fever; it is certainly not the only one.[72]

[464] Professor Schmidt refuses to believe that cadaverous miasma can be carried by the examining fingers of the students in Berlin simply because the same fingers do not occasion childbed fever among all those who deliver normally. I find it impossible to suppress my wonder at this. Professor Schmidt says, "Since September 1844, when the medical direction of the maternity hospital was entrusted to me, until May 1850, of 2,631 patients 442 have been transferred to other stations. Seven died in the first five days after birth and 6 died in the maternity hospital after a longer period of time. Every patient is transferred as soon as her health becomes doubtful. This seems to be the reason why the great destroying angel of the maternity hospitals appears so seldom in the Charité."[73] Professor Schmidt sends 442 of 2,631 patients to other stations, and in spite of the misfortune of so many hundreds of patients, Professor Schmidt does not notice that those who deliver normally contract puerperal fever. The reader knows that in consequence of unavoidable self-infection less than 1 patient from 100 dies. Thus, of 2,631 patients, at

72. Joseph Hermann Schmidt, "Die geburtshülflich-klinischen Institute der königlichen Charité," *Annalen des charité-Krankenhauses zu Berlin* 1(1850), [485–523]: 498–501 [author's note].

73. Ibid., pp. 491f. [author's note].

most 25 would die from self-infection. In the hospital, 13 patients died. How many died of the 442 who were transferred to other stations? The death of so many patients was not sufficient to enable Professor Schmidt to realize that the destroying angel has also reaped a rich harvest in the Charité. . . .

[465–67] [The following passage is from a short letter Semmelweis received from Dr. D. Everken, director of the Paderborn maternity clinic.]

I must admit that one circumstance, which you have identified in your communication as the cause [of childbed fever], did occur simultaneously with the outbreak of the disease. From time to time in the morgue I dissected those corpses associated with the maternity hospital. I could not imagine that this circumstance is the universal cause, but I was led [by your communication] to avoid undertaking any procedures on maternity patients after examining corpses. Thereafter there was no more puerperal fever. I must add that a short time later, while the disease was still spreading, the maternity hospital was separated from the general hospital. From that time on not even sporadic cases have been observed. You must admit, Herr colleague, that it is difficult to judge; perhaps nowhere outside medicine is one more readily deceived by *post hoc ergo propter hoc* reasoning.[74]

[468] Rudolf Virchow says, in his *Collected Papers on Scientific Medicine*, "Explorers of nature recognize no bugbears other than individuals who speculate."[75] Boër formulated the same truth as follows: "If every century could produce one physician as observant (as Hippocrates) rather than so many who are educated in theoretical systems, how much more would have been achieved for humanity and for animal life generally."[76] Boër, the author

74. Paderborn, 17 February 1858 [author's note].
75. Rudolf Virchow, *Gesammelte Abhandlungen zur wissenschaftlichen Medicin* (Frankfurt am Main: [Meidinger and Sohn], 1856), p. 737 [author's note].
76. Rogers Lucas Johann Boër, *Abhandlungen und Versuche zur Begrundung einer neuen, einfachen und naturgemässen Geburtshülfe* (Vienna: von Mösk, 1810), vol. 2, p. 3

of seven books on natural obstetrics, had a right to speak in this way. But Virchow, who because of his many speculations is himself a bugbear for the exploration of nature, Virchow who is such a poor observer that as a pathological anatomist he is not yet able to detect resorption in corpses of patients who die of childbed fever, Virchow has no right to speak like this, unless, of course, in a moment of jovial honesty Virchow was characterizing himself.

[469] Naturally, in this essay we must restrict ourselves to Virchow's speculations about puerperal fever. Virchow's claim that natural science knows no bugbears other than persons who speculate is submerged in a mass of speculation. It appears, in fact, in the introduction to an unsuccessful attempt to depict puerperal fever. In this introduction Virchow speaks of menstruation, conception, and pregnancy as phenomena that relate causally to puerperal fever. The anatomist, the surgeon, a person treated surgically, the male or female infant who dies of puerperal fever—who dies from pyemia in my sense—has never menstruated, has never conceived, was never pregnant, but nevertheless dies of the same disease that kills the maternity patients. Moreover, my theory, which teaches how to restrict puerperal fever to less than 1 percent, is not based on the prevention of menstruation, conception, or pregnancy. Pregnancy provides nothing more than a resorbant surface. But in anatomists, surgeons, those operated upon, and newborn infants, pregnancy provides no such surface and puerperal fever originates nevertheless. Among maternity patients, the resorbant surface does not cause puerperal fever unless that surface is contaminated with decaying matter. How inconsequential the inner surface of the uterus is for the origin of childbed fever follows from the fact that the same opportunity is provided by the smallest injury in any location of either the female or male body.

[470] Virchow says, "Two circumstances are important for the occurrence of puerperal fever epidemics: weather conditions and simultaneous illness. In the first respect it appears that the largest number of epidemics occur in winter months. To simultaneous illnesses belong, in addition to acute exanthemata, well

developed cases of erysipelas, croup, and discharging or infected inflammations."[77] It is entirely true that the largest number of epidemics occur in winter, but this is not because of weather conditions. Rather it is because winter is particularly the time when there is contact with decaying matter. . . . It is equally correct that puerperal fever appears at the same time as acute exanthemata, developed cases of erysipelas, etc., and the cause of the simultaneous appearance is that such diseases are treated by physicians and midwives—the same persons who also treat maternity patients.

If the tables I have provided in this book do not convince Virchow, then I counsel him to request that the Minister of Education abolish all instruction in obstetrics during the winter months. This could be done for as many years as it takes to convince Virchow that winter weather does not cause epidemics of childbed fever. I do not regard as valid the objection that it is impossible to interrupt obstetrical training in this way. In the first place, Virchow has shown himself to be a wretched observer in matters relating to puerperal fever. But ignoring this, any obstetrical training that would enable him to make such observations in a lecture in 1858 at a meeting of the Society for Obstetrics in Berlin without a single voice having been raised against him, any such obstetrical training is so entirely worthless that its suppression can only be an advantage. *[471]* How could the obstetrical training in Berlin be other than worthless if Professor Schmidt believes in a nosocomial atmosphere? . . .

As a physiological condition, puerperal thrombosis [blood clots remaining fixed at the site of origin and causing vascular obstruction] exists only in Virchow's speculation and certainly not in the uteruses of patients. *[472]* As a pathological condition puerperal thrombosis is created when blood disintegrates after the resorption of decaying matter. As a pathological condition puerperal thrombosis is a localization of disintegrated blood just like peritonitis, endometritis, etc. Virchow believes that after loss of the placenta the contractions of the uterus are not sufficient to prevent hemorrhage and that physiological puerperal thrombo-

77. Virchow, op. cit., note 75 above, p. 779.

sis completely closes the vascular system. The contractions of the uterus are themselves entirely sufficient to prevent hemorrhage; through the contractions, not only are the vascular lumina restricted, but simultaneously the uterus is shortened longitudinally so that the length of the veins is reduced. In this way the course of the vascular system is restricted. The walls of the vascular system are so convoluted that upon contraction the vessels completely close. This takes place unless the blood is thinned by high temperature; given such a temperature, the patient bleeds to death.

Puerperal thrombosis does not exist as a physiological condition. This is proven by dissections, although Virchow also appeals to dissections to prove that it exists. We will now determine who is correct. If a patient dies without having had puerperal fever, one never finds a thrombus in her uterus; if a patient dies of puerperal fever one may or may not find thrombosis as a product of the disintegrated blood. But even if one finds thrombosis, so many vessels may be free that from these [if Virchow were correct,] the patient would have bled to death.

[473] Because physiological puerperal thrombosis does not exist, puerperal fever cannot be caused when thrombi decay into ichor. [Moreover,] I can prove that puerperal fever does not originate in this way, since my teachings, which restrict puerperal fever to less than 1 patient in 100, do not prevent physiological thrombosis or the decay of thrombi into ichor. To prove that physiological thrombosis leads to puerperal fever Virchow says: "The better the uterus contracts, the better are the conditions for the uterine-vascular system; conversely, the danger is always somewhat greater when contraction is not complete. The best observers agree that in metrophlebitis the uterus normally remains slightly enlarged."[78] In metrophlebitis the uterus certainly remains enlarged, but enlargement is the effect, not the cause, of metrophlebitis. . . . Imperfect contraction does not lead to physiological thrombosis and this in turn to puerperal fever. Rather, since metrophlebitis can be prevented by chlorine washing, inadequate contraction follows from metrophlebitis and this

78. Ibid., p. 599.

follows from disintegration of the blood. *[474]* By washing in chlorine one destroys decaying matter that would cause puerperal fever. How could washing the hands prevent physiological thrombosis or the metamorphosis of thrombi?

What ridiculous things are recommended when the majority write about things they do not understand. Virchow believes that the better the contractions the less the danger that physiological thrombosis will lead to puerperal fever. Moreover, he says, good contractions

> apparently occur after an exceptional shock to the nerves, and it may be that timely lactation or, occasionally, milk fever has a great influence in this respect. All paralyzing and weakening influences, which greatly retard contractions of the uterus, also hinder contraction of the vascular system. Perhaps this explains, too, why those who deliver in confinement and so receive such a shock to their nervous systems, so seldom become dangerously ill, while in spite of the best treatment, weak patients so often die, especially in the overfilled maternity hospitals where they are under miasmatic influences.[79]

Thus Virchow believes that lactation and great nervous excitement protect one against puerperal fever. *[475]* [By contrast] Kiwisch writes, "I have learned that during epidemics non-nursing mothers become ill significantly less often than those who nurse. Thus at the Prague hospital more patients became ill among paying patients who did nurse than among those who did not."[80] Scanzoni finds nervous excitement to be the cause of the greater mortality at the training institute for obstetricians, and Professor Braun agrees. . . .

[476–77] . . . Not to mention those of my students who are physicians and surgeons, 823 of my students are now midwives practicing in Hungary. These know better than Virchow why the largest number of puerperal epidemics occur in winter, and what must be done to avoid simultaneous puerperal fever and erysipelas, croup, ichorous and purulent infections. They are more enlightened than the members of the Society for Obstetrics in

79. Ibid., p. 600.
80. Kiwisch, op. cit., note 47 above, p. 625.

Berlin; they would laugh Virchow to scorn if he attempted to lecture them on epidemic puerperal fever.[81]

[478] [Semmelweis now reprints an essay entitled "Toward an Examination of the Causes of Puerperal Fever" by Anselm Martin, director of the Munich Maternity Hospital.]

A lamentable misfortune for the recently erected Munich maternity hospital has been the appearance of an epidemic of puerperal fever that, with brief intermissions, raged from the middle of December 1856 until the end of June 1857. From 1 October until the end of July, 1,090 patients were cared for; of these, 88 became ill of puerperal fever or related pathological disorders, and 37 died. . . .

One usually cites unfavorable location, overcrowding, uncleanliness, etc. as the most important causes; now, however, the suffering has appeared in a building entirely new from the ground up, entirely dry and clean, and one pronounced habitable by sanitation and building officials. Light and air are accessible everywhere; the whole spacious building is newly equipped and furnished. Each maternity ward holds only six beds, and these beds are changed regularly. Whole wings of the large building are often left empty and locked up, all the beds are then cleaned and the whole wing generally aired out. *[479]* Every possible cause of the disease was anticipated and circumvented with the utmost care. All who are sick in any way are immediately taken to the general hospital; only the few who can no longer be transferred are cared for in the maternity ward.

Corpses are removed within a few hours. The sick are given special treatment in a separate and appropriately located room. The service personnel for the sick are not allowed to visit healthy patients, and they do not live with the other personnel. Laundry for the sick is cleaned separately and carefully, and reused only after thorough airing. Syringes, catheters, etc. for the sick are used only in sick rooms and are always cleaned carefully and stored

---

81. Some of Semmelweis's biographers have taken this remark as evidence that by the time Semmelweis wrote the *Ätiologie* he was already losing his grip on reality. György Gortvay and Imre Zoltán, *Semmelweis: His Life and Work* (Budapest: Akadémiai Kiadó, 1968), pp. 185f. It is difficult to see how the remark can have been interpreted in this way, given that it is unquestionably true.

separately. Physicians who visit ill patients are required to wash in chlorine water as they leave the sick room. In regimen, cleanliness, diet, etc. all those cared for throughout the entire hospital are diligently supervised day and night, and are watched hourly. Physicians who visited the hospital during the epidemic and who saw all these arrangements and the regulation and supervision could not believe that this institution, whose circumstances were unrivaled and incapable of improvement, could have an epidemic of puerperal fever. . . .

[480] . . . Epidemic puerperal fever is already thoroughly discussed in the literature; it is not our intention to present variations in what is already well known. In spite of this literature, the disease is not less common, its statistics more encouraging, or therapy more successful. It may be the obligation of larger maternity hospitals occasionally to report facts that appear in the quest for possible causes. Experience in this area is still deficient. . . . We therefore present a few preliminary contributions for the further investigation of etiological factors from the newly constructed Munich maternity hospital.[82] . . .

The time is past for further exploration of the etiological factors of childbed fever, since the universal etiological factor for all cases without a single exception has been discovered in decaying animal-organic matter. The time has now come to make harmless this universal etiological factor in order that throughout the whole world the disease will be less common, its statistics more encouraging, and its therapy more successful in the sense that the therapy has no opportunity to be unsuccessful. . . .

[481] . . . Infection from cadavers is sometimes identified as a cause of puerperal fever, particularly at maternity hospitals. The cadaverous particles that adhere to the hands of physicians and students after examinations or exercises on corpses, or the cadaverous smell that is retained after washing with soap and water, supposedly generates putrid air that, upon penetration, causes puerperal processes. Even the smell of corpses adhering to cloth-

82. Anselm Martin, "Zur Erforschung der Ursachen des epidemischen Puerperalfiebers," *Monatsschrift für Geburtskunde und Frauenkrankheiten* 10 (1857), [253–73: 253f.; author's note].

ing, linen, etc. is supposed to cause this infection. Although supported by many, this cause has yet to be accepted by science. Without wishing to prejudice the issue either way, we believe it necessary to mention the following facts.

[482] After having no occurrences of the disease through January and February, two patients suddenly became ill on the same day with what appeared to be epidemic puerperal fever. Both delivered normally on the same day and almost at the same hour. In neither case could a single factor in the entire building be identified that could have been the cause. We finally discovered that, unknown to the authorities of the institution, an assistant had autopsied an infant corpse in a remote dissection room, washed carefully with chlorine water, and immediately thereafter examined the two patients. Because the patients became ill unusually soon after delivery, and because only these two from the entire hospital became ill, the guilty person admitted the facts. He also admitted that the same thing occurred in December, on the day when puerperal fever first appeared in the hospital. At that time, the first patients to become ill were those he examined immediately after opening a corpse.

In December and in the middle of February, possibly by cadaverous infection, several other cases of puerperal fever occurred. It spread quickly through the hospital. This was always accompanied by a general sickliness of the patients and it required a space of sixteen to twenty-one days before circumstances improved. It may be appropriate to add that the university obstetrical clinic of the Munich maternity hospital is held daily from ten until eleven in the morning. A great number of practicing physicians attend this immediately after attending a medical clinic that is filled with persons suffering from typhoid. Many others come from the anatomy hall, so that in the air of the delivery room and the maternity ward the smell of the anatomy ward is detectable. Moreover, so many practitioners handle corpses during autopsies that it is impossible to supervise and correct this situation.

[483] Only while the university obstetrical clinic is open and only since it has been connected with the Munich maternity hospital (since 1824) do the records contain descriptions of outbreaks of epidemic puerperal fever. The earlier records, although very exact, hardly mention this disease. Practitioners who live in the building often undertake studies in microscopical or chemical

pathological anatomy, and from these they are often called quickly to examine women in labor. Exact supervision of these examinations is also impossible. All these circumstances, added to other precarious features, also were present in the earlier location without the appearance of epidemic puerperal fever.

In consequence of a royal decree, the university obstetrical clinic was closed from the beginning of April until 22 June. The disease did not end completely, but was less frequent and less serious. With the beginning of a better season in June, the disease ended completely. In July, as the clinic was again visited by students, rapid and fatal cases of the disease appeared. They ended as the semester closed and the clinic was no longer visited by students. One must not assume that in these cases there was infection by the students. *[484]* The cases occurred sporadically, as is common at the close of an epidemic.[83]

These observations speak so loudly for themselves that they require no comment. Although this was not made explicit, students were required to wash in chlorine water before examinations. The maternity hospital in Munich is a striking proof that, in spite of excellent accommodations, complete prevention is impossible unless all governments strictly administer the previously mentioned law—namely, that everyone who is occupied in a maternity hospital is forbidden from contacting decaying matter. Is it fair to make the safety of maternity hospitals dependent on the goodwill of students? Even with the best intentions, can it not happen that great evil will be provoked through the carelessness of a few?

Carl Braun was my successor as assistant and is currently Professor of Obstetrics at the first clinic in Vienna, the very clinic whose striking data enabled me to discover that the previously accepted etiology of childbed fever was false, and where I discovered the eternally true etiology of the disease. Braun opposes the etiology that I have discovered.[84] These circumstances may

83. Ibid., pp. 259–61.
84. Here Semmelweis cites Braun, op. cit., note 24 above, p. 465. In this passage Braun refers to Jakob Henle's suggestion that microorganisms may be causally responsible for various diseases. Semmelweis never discussed the pos-

incline the reader to give Braun's judgment greater weight than that of my other opponents. I am, therefore, obliged to refute him somewhat more fundamentally. However, Carl Braun makes this easy; he says in rapid succession things so entirely nonsensical that I must be cautious to avoid suspicion that I have distorted his position. Therefore, I cannot simply mention his main objections as I have done with other opponents; to escape this suspicion I must cite him word for word. . . .

[485–88] . . . According to Carl Braun there are thirty causes of childbed fever. The twenty-eighth of these is cadaverous infection. Of this he says the following:

> In 1847 Semmelweis sought to establish this as the leading, almost the only cause of epidemics of puerperal fever. According to this theory, cadaverous particles adhere to the hands after examinations or exercises on corpses. Even after washing with soap and water, the remaining smell or putrid vapor initiates puerperal processes when introduced in internal examinations of patients. Semmelweis found a defender in Professor Skoda. . . .
>
> *[489]* . . . Semmelweis bases his opinion on the following [seven] claims [lettered (a) through (g) and widely spread over the next several pages]: (a) Mortality is higher in the Viennese school for obstetricians, with its pathological examinations, than in the school for midwives. (b) When physicians wash their hands with a solution of chlorinated lime before examining patients, the cadaverous smell no longer remains on the hands, and patients are protected against those puerperal processes that otherwise follow obstetrical examinations.

Braun objects to these two claims as follows:

> During the winter of 1849 there was an epidemic of puerperal fever at the first clinic in spite of the required use of chlorine washings. Without an ascertainable [*eruirbare*] cause this epidemic ended in April when the weather improved. Although Professor Klein, director of the clinic, continued to instruct without interruption, and although the assistant industriously undertook op-

---

sibility that microorganisms could be the cause of puerperal fever, but since he had read Braun's passage he must at least have been aware of that possibility.

erations on cadavers with students, among 1,818 patients there were only 29 fatalities, that is, 1.5 percent. *[490]* In the winter semester 1849–50, puerperal fever became more prevalent as was usual in the fall. Of 1,888 births there were 77 deaths (2 percent [actually 4.08 percent]). These occurrences must seriously weaken belief in the effectiveness of calcium chloride.

Following Semmelweis's lecture, a chlorine solution was made available in an open bowl in which all the students washed their hands; they also cleaned them with a nail brush.[85] This disinfectant solution smelled only faintly of chlorine and the sediment contained progressively more gypsum. For these reasons an enclosed glass canister was brought into the delivery room; fresh chlorine solution was added before the rounds and the solution was drawn off through an attached pipette. Before or after every examination each student washed with clean, abundantly chlorinated water. From January until March this continual and most conscientious disinfection of all the examiners' hands was accompanied by an increase in the epidemic from 3.9 percent to 5 percent. With the end of the summer semester of 1850, puerperal processes ceased, so that from 1,725 births only 10 deaths occurred (.5 percent). Because corpses decay much more quickly in summer than in winter, and the smell of corpses is retained longer on the hands of those who carry out operational exercises, it was observed that this smell was not destroyed after frequent handling of patients and of cleaning with chlorine solution . . . We no longer trusted blindly in the disinfective power of the chlorine solution when used in the accepted way. Each student was required conscientiously to abstain from examining patients if he had touched corpses on the same day. *[491]* Irrespective of the greatest caution, puerperal fever claimed from 3 to 5 percent in January and [through?] December 1851, and indeed in March 7.2 percent.

Through the years of 1849 to 1852, as no doubt in all earlier times, all known measures were employed with the greatest caution. At the school for midwives, infection from corpses is certainly not easily possible; moreover, chlorine washing had been strictly supervised, there had been a cautious director and an experienced assistant, and there were no ascertainable changes in

---

85. Semmelweis seems to have introduced use of the nail brush as a means of futhering disinfection. Gortvay and Zoltán, op. cit., note 81 above, p. 52.

other circumstances. Nevertheless, in January and March of 1852, from 10 to 12 percent of the patients died tragically of puerperal fever. These facts weaken the hypothesis of cadaverous infection—an hypothesis that draws very bold conclusions primarily from the past—and admonish us to consider other etiological factors. A surgeon could not form an adequate opinion if suddenly told that all cases of pyemia and hospital infection among his patients through the course of many years were due to his pupils who practiced on cadavers. No more could an obstetrician make an instantaneous judgment regarding all the different influences that affected the health of a maternity hospital over several decades.[86] . . .

[492–94] . . . We have seen that Braun contests [the hypothesis of] cadaverous infections while still seeking protection [for his patients] from cadaverous infection. We find the same contradiction regarding calcium chloride—he denies that it has any disinfective properties, but he also teaches a more perfect method of using it. In 1848 I employed the disinfective properties of calcium chloride in an imperfect way and had only 10 preventable cases of infection from without. Braun, with an improved method for exploiting the disinfectant, had 65, 37, 34, 137, and 52 preventable deaths from infections between 1849 and 1853. *[495]* In spite of a more perfect method, Braun had more cases of infection. This is because his opposition to my teachings causes students to be negligent.

How competent Braun is to speak on the etiology of childbed fever epidemics is revealed in his view that epidemics originate without ascertainable changes and cease without an ascertainable cause. Nevertheless, he knows thirty causes of childbed fever. Scanzoni allowed only some of his patients to die of childbed fever without an ascertainable cause; for the rest he found a reliable etiological factor in chance.

While I functioned as assistant, chlorine washings were not used in the second clinic. Braun claims that in 1849 they were used and strictly supervised. The strictness of the supervision is revealed in the mortality rates. In the first clinic, as a result of

86. Braun, op. cit., note 24 above, pp. 472–74.

the washings, the rate sank from 9.92 percent to 3.57 percent; in the second clinic at the same time the rate was reduced from 3.35 percent to 3.06 percent. The highly experienced assistant who strictly supervised the chlorine washings at the second clinic, and who nevertheless had a mortality rate of 10 percent in January and 12 percent in March 1852, was Dr. Späth, currently Professor of Obstetrics at Joseph Academy in Vienna. I do not mention Dr. Späth to defame him through association with such a great mortality, but rather because the reader must believe what I am saying about this highly experienced assistant in order to become convinced that what I say is true.

[496] Anyone familiar with obstetrical literature knows that Dr. Späth has carried out work during which his hands would become contaminated with decaying matter. I doubt that, as an opponent of my theories, he would strictly supervise or himself strictly observe the chlorine washings. This suggests the possibility of infection, and what we have hereby shown to be possible Chiari reports to be actual. After reporting how puerperal epidemics occurred twice in the Prague maternity clinic because the genitals of two patients became gangrenous, Chiari says, "Also at the local clinic for midwives a similar observation was made this fall as my friend Dr. Späth has confidentially reported."[87] Braun says that infection from corpses is not easily possible at the school for midwives but Dr. Zipfl has totally refuted him.

Braun says that 7 percent mortality at the first clinic and 12 percent at the second during use of chlorine washings weakens the hypothesis of infection from cadavers, and leads him to consider other etiological factors. He has cast about and come up with an additional twenty-nine causes for childbed fever. We will later demonstrate that the majority of these factors are really not etiological factors and that the others are causes precisely because they provide opportunity for decaying matter either to be generated internally or to be conveyed from external sources. *[497]* For me these facts do not challenge the hypothesis of ca-

87. Baptist Johann Chiari, "Winke zur Vorbeugung der Puerperal-Epidemie," *Wochenblatt der Zeitschrift der k. k. Gesellschaft der Ärzte zu Wien* 11(1855), 117–21: 119.

daverous infection; on the contrary they strengthen it. It speaks for the truth of the hypothesis if its opponents have a greater mortality rate than do those who adopt it. For opponents are not as conscientious in their use of chlorine washings as are those who believe in cadaverous infection. . . .

[498] . . . "(c) When ichor or exudation originating from female or male corpses of those who died from the most diverse diseases is introduced into the uterus of a rabbit that has just given birth, fatal pyemia often results. Often, however, week-long brushing of the surface of the puerperal uterus is not damaging to the rabbit; the animal remains healthy, conceives after the experiment is concluded, and delivers living young." *[499]* Braun responds to this as follows:

> Experiments on animals demonstrate that injections of ichor or brushing the uterus with various exudations is often, but not always, fatal; in dissections, pyemia can be demonstrated. These experiments are certainly carried out differently from the way in which maternity patients are supposedly infected with cadaverous matter. They also raise the question whether mishandling of animals after delivery cannot itself produce death and the results obtained in dissection. The introduction of ichor is often not fatal, and experienced veterinarians, Hayne and others, have established that among domesticated animals puerperal fever often occurs spontaneously in large numbers.[88]

When Carl Braun admits that dissections of rabbits disclose pyemia, he has admitted all that I intended this experiment to prove, namely, that childbed fever is the same disease that arises when decaying matter is introduced into the organism. . . .

[500] . . . "(d) Puerperal fever epidemics occur only in maternity hospitals and never outside." Braun responds as follows:

> History speaks clearly on the spread of puerperal fever epidemics in different countries and cities, over flat lands and on the highest mountains, and it is the current experience of practicing obstetricians that this feared disease occurs in the most diverse social circles. This leaves no doubt in the matter [that the disease occurs epi-

---

88. Braun, op. cit., note 24 above, pp. 465f and 474.

demically outside hospitals]. However, statistical information on the occurrence of lethal puerperal processes in private homes is difficult to obtain, partly because these deaths are reported in newspapers under other names such as nervous fever, typhoid, paralysis of the lungs, etc. This is partly because in many countries, such as Austria, humane laws forbid public disclosure of the cause of deaths occurring during birth and from certain female diseases such as carcinoma.[89]

[501] . . . I definitely agree with Braun that puerperal fever epidemics occur in the most varied countries and cities, over flat lands and on the highest mountains, and that one encounters the disease in the most diverse social circles, and why not? Braun trains 150 to 200 obstetricians annually. How thoroughly Braun's students understand the prevention of puerperal fever is proved by 367 preventable deaths by infection in six years [when Carl Braun was associated with the first maternity clinic] and by 717 preventable deaths by infection in the four years that Gustav Braun, Carl Braun's student, was the assistant there. Dr. Späth trains 260 to 300 midwives at the midwife school each year; how thoroughly Späth's students understand the prevention of puerperal fever is proved by the 12 percent mortality rate in March 1852. Dr. Späth communicated privately to his friend Chiari how puerperal fever originates; but what one communicates privately to one's friends one does not share with students. Thus infectors are trained for various countries and cities, for the flat lands and the highest mountains, and for the most diverse social circles. . . .
[502] "(e) The seasons exert no influence on the origin of puerperal fever." Against this Braun says, "The seasons and related local circumstances exert an influence on puerperal processes that is not the most significant but that is not negligible either. In Vienna the winter semester never has results as favorable as the summer semester, and in other areas and in foreign maternity hospitals one finds similar results."[90] I have proved that seasons have no influence on the origin of childbed fever. . . . *[503]* . . . "(f) Puerperal fever occurs less frequently in so-called street births.

89. Ibid., pp. 466 and 474f.
90. Ibid., pp. 466 and 475.

[To this Braun responds that] in Vienna, among street births the incidence of puerperal fever is no greater than among those who spend months before delivery in the maternity hospital."[91] . . . The reader remembers that I was not allowed to derive from the official reports numerical proof that those who deliver on the street became ill less often than those who deliver in the clinic. Carl Braun, who was assistant for nearly five years, had the opportunity to obtain this proof. He did not do so, and is content simply to deny that women who deliver on the street are healthier. . . .

[504] . . . "(g) Apparently, maternity hospitals in which midwives are trained and in which cadaverous infection is less likely have fewer deaths than those in which physicians are trained." Against this Braun says,

> We deny that in the largest maternity hospital in the world, where 223,868 patients and their infants have received absolutely free care from the state, there is an unusually high mortality rate. At the Vienna free clinic, which has never been closed because of puerperal fever, the mortality rate averages 3.8 percent (5.9 percent in the school for physicians and 3.2 percent in the school for midwives). At the Maternité in Paris, where male students are not accepted, it is 4.1 percent, in Dubois's Clinic 5.6 percent, in the Hospital Beaujou where there is no instruction 16 percent. *[505]* Irrespective of whether physicians or midwives are trained, British hospitals have a lower rate, German hospitals are similar, and Scandinavian hospitals have a higher rate.
>
> Moreover, one must consider that in the Viennese clinic for physicians one encounters not only lethal puerperal processes but also such acute diseases as eclampsia, pneumonia, meningitis, apoplexy, etc., studies of which are important for physicians; that absolutely all who come must be admitted, even diseased women who have just been released from the general hospital; that there are admissions of patients from fifty-two to seventy more days a year than in the clinic for midwives; that admissions include all the miscarriages from the capital and surrounding area represent-

91. Ibid., pp. 466 and 475. "Pregnant women were admitted into the maternity hospital during different months of pregnancy in order that the students could become familiar with the entire course of pregnancy." Györy, op. cit., note 4 above, p. 66.

ing the poorest classes; that puerperal fever victims are not generally transferred; that during the winter semester—the time of epidemics—the first maternity clinic often accepts 100 to 200 more patients a month than does the school for midwives; that dangerous deliveries, which present a great opportunity for the instruction of physicians, are generally taken into the first clinic; that construction of the first clinic precludes spontaneous ventilation through open doors; that until 1849 the first clinic was much nearer to the sick wards in which over 20,000 patients were cared for annually. These facts easily explain why the school for physicians has a mortality rate a few percent higher. This higher rate need not be regarded as supporting the speculative hypothesis of cadaverous infection.

[506] When all the circumstances are taken into account, we cannot, therefore, endorse the observations made in the Viennese maternity hospital in support of the hypothesis of cadaverous infection. We certainly cannot take handling of corpses as an important cause of puerperal fever epidemics in maternity hospitals. However, we would regard it as the greatest foolhardiness to perform or to allow examinations or operations on maternity patients with hands on which one can still detect the smell of corpses.[92]

In contending that the Viennese maternity hospital does not have an unusually large mortality rate, Carl Braun has become my ally; I also reject the Virchow–[Aloys Constantin Conrad Gustav] Veit accusation that the Viennese maternity hospital has a horrible mortality rate. Mortality in the Viennese maternity hospital is no larger than in other similar hospitals. If hospitals have a lower mortality, the reasons are that such hospitals are often closed for months at a time, which has never been the case in Vienna, or that sick patients are transferred out, which happens in Vienna only rarely. [507] However, when Carl Braun attempts to explain the difference in mortality between the Viennese clinics without the "speculative hypothesis of cadaverous infection," then he finds in me an opponent. [Semmelweis criticizes Braun's attempts to explain the greater mortality in the first clinic. This constitutes a review of much of what has been said

92. Braun, op. cit., note 24 above, pp. 466 and 475–77.

earlier. The discussion concludes as follows:] *[508–22]* . . . Carl
Braun calls attention to various disadvantages which can easily
explain the slightly higher mortality rate of the first clinic. I have
already shown that these unfavorable circumstances could not
explain a difference in the mortality rates of the two clinics [be-
cause they operate with at least equal severity in the second clinic].
And moreover, in spite of these [supposedly] unfavorable circumstances, [under my direction] the first clinic had a lower
mortality rate than the second. . . . This demonstrates with
mathematical certainty that these unfavorable conditions in the
first clinic did not occasion the greater mortality. . . .

[523–24] . . . Braun says, "Since the announcement of the
theory of cadaverous infection, over five years have passed. . . .
We find in the literature no confirmation of the practical applicability of the infection theory; we encounter, in fact, the most
decisive claims and experiences that divest this hypothesis of its
most important supports."[93] Braun claims that in more than five
years the literature contains no confirmation of the practical applicability of the infectious theory; the attentive reader knows
that this is not true. But assume that in five years my opinion
had not been validated in practice; that would still not prove that
my opinion is erroneous. Rather, it would prove only the in-
competence of all those who had the opportunity to confirm my
opinions and who had not done so. *[525]* The practical applicability of my opinion was confirmed during my service in Vienna; this is an eternally true fact. If my opinion were erroneous,
then its practical applicability could not have been demonstrated
during that time. . . . Need discloses one's true friends, and I
was in need because my opinion was nowhere confirmed in
practice; I found my true friend in Carl Braun. For Braun, following me, reduced mortality in the first clinic from 9.92 percent to 2.48 percent. By reducing mortality by 7.44 percent he
has confirmed the practical applicability of my opinions. . . .

[526–29] . . . Having successfully defended the claim that decaying matter is the universal cause of childbed fever, I will now

93. Ibid., pp. 466 and 472.

judge the thirty causes of childbed fever that Braun lists. Many of Braun's purported causes are really not causes at all; the actual causes of childbed fever that he lists are causes only because they generate decaying matter internally or because they convey external decaying matter to the individual. Thus Braun's etiology is partly true and partly false. It is true when he teaches what I teach; it is false when he teaches anything else.

[530] Braun's [purported] etiological factors of childbed fever that are really not causes include the following: (1) conception and pregnancy; (2) hyperinosis; (3) hydremia; (4) uremia [excessive and toxic retention of metabolic by-products in the blood]; (5) universal plethora; (6) a disproportion in the vegetation of the mother and fetus; (7) vascular engorgement and stasis [diminution of the flow of blood] caused by pregnancy; (8) whether inopexia of the blood is a cause of puerperal fever remains to be decided; (9) pregnancy fever is not a cause of puerperal fever but is a fever that occurs in pregnancy and is true puerperal fever; (11) the equalization of hyperinosis; (12) inopexia of maternity—this does not exist as a physiological condition; as a pathological condition it is a product of puerperal fever rather than its cause; (13) reduced pressure exerted on adjacent organs because of the shrinking of the uterus; (15) injuring the inner surface of the uterus through separation of the placenta; (16) puerperal thrombosis and metrorrhagia [abnormal uterine bleeding]—as we have seen, puerperal thrombosis does not exist as a physiological condition; as a pathological condition it is an effect, not a cause, of childbed fever. Metrorrhagia is not a cause of childbed fever. Before adoption of chlorine washings puerperal fever usually followed metrorrhagia, thereafter it rarely did so; *[531]* . . . (18) suppression of milk secretion; (20) individuality of the patient; (22) emotional disturbances; (23) mistakes in diet; (26) chilling; and (29) epidemic influences—as a basis for listing epidemic influences Braun knows nothing to cite other than the fact that this has been used as an explanation for the devastations of puerperal fever from ancient times. . . .

[532] After having so firmly established the existence of epidemic influences, [Braun offers] a four-page discussion of contagion, miasma, and infection and of whether or not childbed

fever is contagious. It is a horrible example of the monstrosities that occur when one compiles without understanding. We leave this chaos unexplored.

To those causes that really are causes of childbed fever belong the following: (10) birth itself; (14) protracted labor; (21) operative interventions—delivery, extended labor, and operative intervention can crush the genitals thereby causing the internal generation of decaying matter; (17) interrupted secretion and excretion of lochia. Interrupted secretion is not a cause of childbed fever; however, interrupted excretion can occasion the disease by self-infection; (19) the harmful influence of the dead fetus. Dead fetuses are not a cause of childbed fever; fetuses that die during birth and that convey foulness through the air that is sucked back into the uterus can cause self-infection; (24) according to Carl Braun, persistent thirst can cause puerperal fever. Thirst may stimulate resorption and consequently also resorption of decaying matter in the uterus. This could then foster self-infection; (25) excessively high room temperatures and deficient ventilation bring about childbed fever because excreted puerperal matter decays more rapidly; (27) how swamp air causes puerperal fever is obvious; *[533]* (28) cadaverous infection; (30) various inappropriate circumstances in maternity hospitals exert a powerful influence on the health of patients. Maternity hospitals that are isolated from adjacent buildings and surrounded by spacious gardens have the lowest mortality rate. Internal contact with general hospitals is a disadvantage, thus all maternity hospitals that are built adjacent to general hospitals have higher average mortality rates. Locations filled with decaying matter, such as morgues, the confluence of drainage canals, unclean lavatories, lavatories with inadequate drainage, and lavatories used to dispose of placentas can all occasion epidemics in nearby hospitals.

[Further inappropriate circumstances that can cause childbed fever include] inadequately constructed ventilation systems in maternity hospitals; rooms adjoining one another without a parallel hallway; poorly ventilated passages that lead into rooms on both sides; windows that are too high, immediately next to one another, or directly over the beds of patients; sick wards that are next to or immediately above or below maternity wards; ventilating in winter through open windows or with air that is too cold; failing to place ventilators in the ceilings, or using ventilators that cause a serious draft of cold air; placing patients with puerperal sickness near maternity wards; requiring patients leaving the delivery room to cross cold passages or stairways; rooms for patients that are too large; placing patients in maternity wards so that they deliver sequentially; *[534]* the effluvium of foul excrements, exudations from patients with putrid fever, or puerperal odors generated when numerous patients live together; failure to isolate the sick, or to close off sick wards; free interchange between those attending ill and healthy patients; doctors or midwives who attend healthy patients after they have examined or injected ill patients; common use of laundry, sponges, and basins by both healthy and sick patients; use of laundry over a period of many years and failure either to clean it adequately or to keep it separated from the laundry of general hospitals; infrequently changing mattresses, straw mattresses, or blankets; continuous use of all parts of a maternity hospital; continuous instruction in overfilled hospitals; inadequate supervision of large numbers of students; overcrowding maternity hospitals in winter; unrestricted admission of healthy and ill patients; patients staying months at a time in the hospital; hospitals being filled with single and deprived women; covering patients excessively in the first eight days [after delivery]; storing placentas or the corpses of infants too long or in rooms adjacent to maternity wards; having too few supervising physicians; allowing constant communication between pregnant patients and patients in the general hospital; admitting patients with zymotic illnesses; an inadequate supply of water on upper floors; large numbers of visitors who remain too long or who spend nights in the maternity wards; excessive examination during prolonged deliveries; facilities that are too small; failing to care for patients in private homes and at public cost when overcrowding makes it advantageous to do so; and failure to remove those suffering from puerperal disease. *[535]* These disadvantages explain the success or failure of different hospitals, and they make hospitals more dangerous than private homes. These various local circumstances, which can often be corrected only at great cost, exert a powerful influence on the origin, virulence, and spread of puerperal fever.[94]

94. Ibid., pp. 485–87.

These disadvantages, listed by Carl Braun, are either not causes of childbed fever, or they cause it only by bringing external decaying matter to patients. . . .

I will give Carl Braun's definition of childbed fever because it is yet another example of undigested compilation. *[536]* According to Braun, childbed fever is a zymotic sickness of acute character that is occasioned in strongly predisposed individuals by general traumata, such as emotional shock, chilling, etc., but that is generally due to characteristic influences, such as miasma, contagion, or decaying animal matter, whereby the foreign matter operates as a yeast and through contact with which the blood is made to ferment.[95]

The reader will note with astonishment that Carl Braun, the same Carl Braun who totally rejects the speculative hypothesis of cadaverous infection, who to the satisfaction of every true friend of humanity has successfully restored the unrestricted operation of epidemic influences, has defined puerperal fever in terms of decaying animal matter rather than in terms of epidemic influences. Oh Logic! Oh Logic! In taking leave of our Viennese colleague we recommend most urgently that if he should again feel called upon to fight for the epidemic deaths of maternity patients, he should first attend at least one semester of logic.

95. Ibid., p. 424.

Epilogue

[537] I do not undertake these polemics because of pugnaciousness. My four years of silence prove this. Given the opposition to my beliefs, however, the unbiased reader will agree not only that the time for silence is past but also that I have the right and obligation to engage in these polemics.

When, with my current convictions, I look into the past, I can endure the miseries to which I have been subjected only by looking at the same time into the future; I see a time when only cases of self-infection will occur in the maternity hospitals of the world. In comparison with the great numbers thus to be saved in the future, the number of patients saved by my students and by me is insignificant. If I am not allowed to see this fortunate time with my own eyes, therefore, my death will nevertheless be brightened by the conviction that sooner or later this time will inevitably arrive.

Index

Index

Abandonment of infants, 110

Abortion: 110; attempted, as a cause of childbed fever, 14

Alzheimer's disease, 58

Anatomical: foundations of medicine, 94; orientation of the Vienna medical school, 88, 119, 128, 154; pathology. *See* Pathological anatomy

Anatomists, as victims of childbed fever, 47, 117, 148, 204, 229. *See also* Pyemia, among surgeons and anatomists

Andral, Gabriel, cited, 25*n*

Anemia, reduces incidence of childbed fever, 206

Animal experiments: recommended by Scanzoni, 200; Semmelweis's, criticized by Braun, 241; Semmelweis's, criticized by Scanzoni, 197; undertaken by Semmelweis, 23, 37–38, 105, 173, 181, 190, 216, 227

Animals, diseased or dead, as a source of decaying animal-organic matter, 148

Antiphlogistic treatment, for childbed fever, 14–15, 134, 189

Arneth, Franz Hektor: biographical note, 125*n*; mentioned, 20*n*, 23, 35, 35*n*, 42, 125, 174, 209, 210; publishes accounts of childbed fever cases, 141–47; quoted, 126–27

Atmospheric-cosmic-terrestrial influences: as causes of childbed fever, 199, 200; irrelevant to childbed fever, 66, 121, 126, 128, 132, 139, 155, 188, 204; meaning of phrase, 65, 65*n*, 86; physicians helpless against, 17*n*, 84. *See also* Atmospheric influences; Epidemic influences

Atmospheric influences: as causes of childbed fever, 12, 16, 17, 33, 36*n*, 112, 204, 208; irrelevant to childbed fever, 38, 67, 122–23, 128, 130, 133, 139–41, 152–57 passim, 162. *See also* Atmospheric-cosmic-terrestrial influences; Epidemic influences

Ausculation, Skoda pioneered, 82*n*

Bacteriology, 55. *See also* Germ, theory of disease; Koch, Robert

Bartsch, Franz Xavier, mentioned, 173

Bed linen, unclean, as a cause of childbed fever, 111–13, 116, 162, 195

Bednar, Alois, mentioned, 100

Bender, Dr. in Frankfurt am Main, 217

Berlin: Charité hospital in, 227–28; Obstetrical Society of, 6, 230, 232–33

Bichat, Xavier, mentioned, 26*n*

Birly, Ede Flórián: biographical note, 129*n*; never accepted Semmelweis's views, 24*n*, 56, 129

Blood: composition of, in pregnancy, 204, 206; disintegration of, in childbed fever (*see* Disintegration of the blood, in childbed fever)

Bloodletting: and sexual norms, 5; as a treatment for childbed fever, 14. *See also* Antiphlogistic treatment, for childbed fever

Boër, Rogers Lucas Johann: biographical note, 70*n*; mentioned, 70, 74, 74*n*, 129; quoted, 154–55, 228–29

Braun, Carl: biographical note, 92*n*; mentioned, 9*n*, 42, 53, 56, 56*n*, 77*n*, 92, 105, 130, 232; quoted and discussed, 34, 34*n*, 169–70, 187, 236–49

Braun, Gustav, mentioned, 131, 242

Breisky, August, reviews Semmelweis's *Aetiologie*, 41, 43*n*

Breit, Franz, mentioned, 61, 87, 105

British: awareness of Semmelweis, 35, 54, 176*n*; beliefs about childbed fever, 9–13, 46, 46*n*, 49; cases of childbed fever reported in, medical literature, 144–47; occurrence of childbed fever in, hospitals, 137–40, 152, 156; relation between, and Semmelweis regarding childbed fever, 30, 31, 36–37, 42, 46, 46*n*, 147–50, 174; use of chlorine washings, 53, 139, 212

Brücke, Ernst Wilhelm Ritter von, mentioned, 190, 226

Brydon, a physician reporting on childbed fever in Sicily, 151

Budapest: mentioned, 16, 23, 24, 56, 58, 106; Semmelweis's lectures in, 36*n*, 112*n*. *See also* Pest, maternity clinic; St. Rochus hospital

Bugbears for science, Virchow's comments about, 228–29

Busch, Dietrich Wilhelm Heinrich, mentioned, 226

Cadaverous poison: as a cause of childbed fever, 28–29, 30, 34, 42, 43, 44, 51, 88, 89. 92, 93, 98, 100, 171, 178, 181, 182, 189, 190, 212, 217, 219, 234–35, 237, 239, 244, 245, 247; as the only cause of childbed fever, 20, 20*n*

Caesarean section, childbed fever victim delivered by, 116, 204

Cancer of the uterus, compared with childbed fever, 147. *See also* Carcinoma; Medullary Cancer

Carcinoma: a source of decaying organic matter, 202; in women not publicly disclosed, 242

Carious knee, patient with, a source of

decaying organic matter: discussed, 43–44, 93; mentioned, 106, 114, 116, 117, 119, 171, 185, 193, 194

Causes of disease, general discussions of, 26–28, 37–38, 55, 216. *See also* Childbed fever, cause of

Chance deaths, from childbed fever in Scanzoni's account, 192, 195, 196, 201, 211, 239

Characterizing diseases, methods of, 25–28 passim, 46–48. *See also* Childbed fever, characterizations of

Charité in Berlin, 227–228

Chiari, Johann Baptist: biographical note, 123*n*; discussed, 218–19; mentioned, 49, 123, 124, 139, 210, 213, 240, 242; reports of cases of childbed fever in Prague quoted, 134–36

Childbed fever: during pregnancy, 16, 18, 83, 115–16, 117, 204; French beliefs about, 46*n*, 49, 77*n*, 133; geographical distribution of, 133, 139, 150–52, 241–42; history of, 8, 152–55, 241; in relation to premature deliveries, 40, 82–83, 86, 100–101, 206; in relation to street births, 40, 80–82, 86, 100–101, 196, 206, 242–43; modern name of, 8; seasonal occurrence of, 15, 40; sequential cases of, 83, 86, 93, 101; similar disease among males, 46*n*, 49, 145; spontaneous cases of, 13, 241; sporadic cases of, 12, 29, 83, 236; symptoms of, 8, 71

—among surgeons and anatomists, 19*n*, 47, 117, 148, 204, 229. *See also* Pyemia, among surgeons and anatomists

—among the newborn, 18, 38, 40, 45–47, 49, 77–79, 80, 86, 99–100, 117, 229

—atmospheric factors as causes of. *See* Atmospheric influences

—British beliefs about. *See* British, beliefs about childbed fever

—cause of: 9–14, 18, 24n, 32–38, 41, 48–51, 65–113 passim, 114, 201–2, 224, 229, 237, 239, 240, 246–49; contagions as, 9–14, 83, 117–18, 133, 139, 181, 182, 200, 209, 246, 249; decaying animal-organic matter as, 20, 93–126 passim, 141, 147–54, 161–62, 163; emotional factors as, 12, 14, 31n, 33, 120, 207–8, 211, 246, 249; endemic, 12, 13, 17–18, 29, 30, 37, 45, 69–75, 81, 84–86, 120, 158–62, 208; not demonstrable, 195, 196, 201, 211; not ascertainable, 237, 239

—characterizations of: anatomical, 221, 249; difficult to provide, 9, 9n, 13; Semmelweis's, 20, 38–39, 51, 99, 114, 204; symptomatic, 8, 46–47, 221, 249

—epidemic. *See* Atmospheric-Cosmic-Terrestrial influences; Atmospheric influences; Epidemic influences

—epidemics of, 70, 127, 133, 134, 153–57, 177, 179, 186, 189, 192, 205, 210, 236, 237–39, 241–42

—prophylaxis and therapy of: 178–79, 212; antiphlogistic, 14–15, 15n, 134, 189; not effective, 136, 234; purges as, 129; Semmelweis's, 39, 41n, 57, 163–67, 223. *See also* Chlorine washings; Prophylaxis of disease

—through self-infection. *See* Self-infection

Chilling, as a cause of childbed fever, 83, 161, 246. *See also* Colds, as causes of childbed fever

Chlorina liquida, 89. *See also* Chlorine washings

Chlorine washings: British use of, 53, 139, 212; critics' comments about, 24n, 32–33, 44, 223, 225, 227, 237–38; others' use of, 127, 128, 128n, 135, 176–77, 180, 189, 192–96 passim, 234, 235, 236, 237–41 passim; Semmelweis's use of, 20, 29, 51, 51n,

89, 92–93, 99–101, 103, 107, 116, 119, 123, 130, 137, 154, 155, 165, 173, 179, 203, 218; use of, in surgery, 173, 219

Cholera, compared to childbed fever, 66–67, 84–86

Churchill, Fleetwood, quoted, 146

Climate, childbed fever appears in every, 123, 157. *See also* Seasons; Weather

Clinics, maternity. *See* Maternity clinics

Clothing, contaminated, as a cause of childbed fever, 145–50 passim

Colds, as causes of childbed fever, 75, 83, 120. *See also* Chilling Commissions investigating childbed fever, 17, 22, 82, 83–84, 86, 92, 95–98, 101, 104, 197, 199, 215–16

Conception, as a cause of childbed fever, 76, 161, 229

Confinement births, 123

Copeland, George A., mentioned, 175

Copenhagen: maternity hospital, 180–88; mentioned, 136, 177, 179

Corpses, poison from. *See* Cadaverous poison

Cowpox inoculations, chlorine washings of comparable value, 21, 112, 172, 213

Crede, Carl S. F., reviews Semmelweis's *Aetiologie*, 41

Croup, in relation to childbed fever, 230, 232

Danube river, in relation to incidence of childbed fever, 151–52

Deathtraps, maternity hospitals called, 110, 200, 209, 215

Decaying animal-organic matter, three sources of, 114–15, 136, 185, 194–96, 212–13, 218. *See also* Childbed fever, cause of, decaying animal-organic matter as; Self-infection

Delivery position, as a cause of childbed fever, 18, 87

Diet: as a cause of childbed fever, 14, 17, 33, 75, 120, 161, 211, 246; as a cause of disease generally, 27n

Dietl, József: biographical note, 186n; mentioned, 187, 188; quoted, 186

Dilation, period of, in relation to onset of childbed fever, 76–77, 86, 98–99, 116, 196, 207

Disease: causes of 26–27, 37–38, 79n, 216, 224; characterizations of, 25, 26–28, 38; prophylaxis and therapy of, 27, 28, 186n. *See also under specific diseases in question*

Disintegration of the blood, in childbed fever, 99, 114, 116, 120, 176, 191–92, 197, 203–4, 208, 213

Docent, Semmelweis's petition to be made a, 105–6

Dropsy, reduces incidence of childbed fever, 206

Dublin: maternity hospital, 87, 137, 140, 142–43; mentioned, 156, 175

Dubois, Paul-Antoine: Parisian maternity clinic of, 125; mentioned, 33

Duka, Theodor, 54

Duties of assistants in Viennese first clinic, 98–99, 102, 103

Duncan, M. J., 54

Eclampsia, conducive to childbed fever, 206–7

Effluvia, as a cause of childbed fever, 11, 189, 212, 248. *See also* Miasmata; Nosocomial atmosphere

Egg of Columbus, Semmelweis's theory called an, 32, 45, 223, 223n

Ehrmann, Charles Henri, 126, 127

Emotions, as causes of childbed fever, 12, 14, 31n, 33, 120, 207–8, 211, 246, 249

Endometritis, in relation to childbed fever, 117, 134–35, 147, 165, 191, 202, 203, 213, 230

England and English. *See* British

Enlightenment, influence of, on the rise of hospitals, 3

Epidemic disease, nature of, 12, 12n, 65, 84–86, 121–22, 126

Epidemic influences: 12, 12n, 44, 50, 65–69, 120–23; as causes of childbed fever, 13, 29, 30, 37, 192, 200, 233, 234, 246; irrelevant to childbed fever, 38, 45, 50, 65–69, 81, 84–86, 120–23, 126, 133, 134, 153–57, 202, 204, 211, 239. *See also* Atmospheric-cosmic-terrestrial influences; Atmospheric influences; Childbed fever, epidemics of

Epithelium, protects against decaying organic matter, 115

Erysipelas, in relation to childbed fever, 11, 46n, 145, 145n, 147, 148, 220, 230, 232

Etiological characterizations of disease, 28, 38, 39, 47–48, 55

Etiology of childbed fever. *See* Childbed fever, cause of

Everkin, D., quoted, 34, 228

Exanthemata, in relation to childbed fever, 206, 229, 230

Exciting causes, 79n, 88

Explanatory force, of Semmelweis's theory, 39–40

Fear, as a cause: of childbed fever, 14, 16, 39, 70–71, 79, 159–60, 207; of hydrophobia, 28

Fleischer, Jozsef, 24n, 57

Forceps, use of in delivery, 67, 70n, 74n, 116, 150, 166

Foreign students, as responsible for childbed fever, 84, 101–5 passim

Foundling home, Viennese. *See* Viennese, foundling home

French: beliefs about childbed fever, 46n, 49, 77n; interest in pathological anatomy, 26; obstetricians, 74n; occurrence of childbed fever in, hospitals, 133, 139, 152. *See also under names of specific individuals and hospitals*

Freud, Sigmund, 6

Fumigation, as prophylaxis for childbed fever, 212

Gangrenous genitals, patients with, 113, 113n, 148–49

Gastric fever, 80

Genius epidemicus, 192, 192n, 195,

Germ: of childbed fever, 101; theory of disease, 5, 236n. *See also* Bacteriology; Koch, Robert

German: 243; obstetricians, 74n, 174; occurrence of childbed fever in, hospitals, 133, 139, 243. *See also under names of specific individuals and hospitals*

Glacis of Vienna, 80, 80n

Graz maternity hospital, 214–15

Haller, Carl: mentioned, 22, 22n, 36n; quoted, 172–73

Hamernik, Joseph, quoted and discussed, 37–38, 215–17

Hayne, Anton, 33, 42n, 210, 241

Hebra, Ferdinand Ritter von: biographical note, 170n; mentioned, 19n, 21, 30, 34, 36n, 42, 57; quoted, 170–72

Helm, Theodor, mentioned, 31n, 50, 152, 210

Henle, Jakob, mentioned, 236n

Herzfelder, Heinrich, mentioned, 32n, 210

Hippocrates: describes childbed fever, 152, 154–55, 228; mentioned, 112

Hirsch, August, as sympathetic to Semmelweis, 41n

Hodge, Hugh Lennox, cited, 151

Holmes, Oliver Wendell: beliefs about childbed fever, 10–13; mentioned, 3, 7, 40, 43n

Hospital Beaujou, 243

Hospital infection, 239

Hôtel-Dieu in Paris, 152–53

Hulme, occurrence of childbed fever in, 144

Hydremia, as a cause of childbed fever, 76, 161, 246

Hydrophobia, 25–28 passim

Hyperinosis, as a cause of childbed fever, 76, 161, 191, 204, 213, 246

Hysteria, as a women's disease, 5–6

Immorality, as a cause of childbed fever, 13, 73, 160, 160n

Individuality of patient, as a cause of childbed fever, 76, 161, 205, 211, 246

Infancy, childbed fever in. *See* Newborn, childbed fever among the

Infanticide, 110

Infected wound diseases, 55n, 56n

Inopexia, as a cause of childbed fever, 76, 246

Internal generation, of decaying animal-organic matter. *See* Self-infection

Ireland, occurrence of childbed fever in, 133, 139, 156. *See also* Dublin

Jenner, Edward, his contribution compared with that of Semmelweis, 21, 112, 172, 213

Joseph Academy in Vienna, 240

Kehrer, Ferdinand Adolph, 35–36

Kiel: maternity hospital, 129, 177–179; mentioned, 137, 172

Kiwisch, Franz, von Rotterau: biographical note, 165n; mentioned, 31, 165, 179, 203, 209; quoted and discussed, 9n, 211–12, 219–21, 232

Klein, Johann: biographical note, 61n; mentioned, 22, 24n, 42, 50, 50n, 54, 61, 82, 82n, 92n, 124n, 154, 173, 184, 197, 237

Koch, Robert, 55, 55n, 56n, 183n

Kolletschka, Jakob: case of, recounted, 18–19, 87–88; mentioned,

Kolletschka, Jakob (*continued*)
20, 38, 45, 89, 117, 148, 149, 217;
pathological remains in, compared
with those in maternity patients, 46,
47, 88, 197–98; quoted, 126*n*

Labor, protracted, as a cause of childbed
fever, 207, 211, 247
Lateral deliveries, 18, 87
Laundry processes, in relation to
childbed fever, 75, 111–13, 116, 136,
233
Lautner, George Marie, mentioned, 105
Laws: prevent disclosure of women's
diseases, 242; to insure cleanliness of
medical personnel, 163–64, 169, 184,
236
Lebert, Hermann, quoted and discussed, 33, 221
Leeches, use of, in treating childbed
fever, 15*n*
Lesky, Erna, 19*n*, 22, 48–49, 51–53
Leukorrhea, mentioned, 5
Levy, Karl Edouard Marius: mentioned, 30*n*, 45; quoted and discussed, 179–88; reports on maternity hospitals in London and Dublin,
136–40
Liebig, Justus, quoted and discussed,
35, 217–18
Light, nature of, 224
Lister, Joseph: Semmelweis's influence
on, 53–55; mentioned, 3, 7
Litzmann, Conrad Theodor: mentioned, 152; quoted 150–51, 178–79
Lochial discharge: 8, 200; irregularities
in, as a cause of childbed fever, 13,
76, 247
Logic, 224, 249
Lumpe, Eduard: mentioned, 9*n*, 12*n*,
40, 45, 46, 49, 53, 209, 210; quoted
and discussed, 223–25; response to
Semmelweis's May 15 lecture, 32–
33; views on childbed fever, 13–16
Lymphangitis, 87, 88, 149, 204

Magendie, François, 217
Markusovszky, Lajos, 4*n*, 23, 36*n*, 54–
55, 74*n*
Martin, Anselm, quoted and discussed, 233–36
Maternité in Paris: described, 125–26;
mentioned, 128, 156, 171
Maternity clinics: conditions in, 4, 69–
70, 74–75, 106–13, 127, 152–53, 174,
218, 243*n*; establishment of, 3;
women's fear of, 4, 69, 70–71
—First and second, in Vienna: 63–64,
94–95, 128, 149–50, 236, 243; differences between, 69–87 passim;
mortality rates in, 16, 17, 20, 28–
29, 40, 50, 51, 64–65, 92, 94–95
—References to specific non-Viennese:
Copenhagen, 180–188; Dublin, 87,
137, 140, 142–43; Dubois's Paris
Clinic, 125, 243; Graz, 214–15; Hôtel-Dieu in Paris, 152–53; Kiel, 129,
177–79; Maternité in Paris, 125–26,
128, 171, 243; Munich, 233–36;
Paderborn, 34, 228; Pest, 62, 106–
13, 115, 116, 129, 130, 148, 154, 195,
213; Prague, 191–214 passim, 232,
240; Strasbourg, 69, 126–29, 156;
Würzburg, 165–66
May 15 lecture, by Semmelweis: account of, 32–35, 210; mentioned,
19*n*, 23, 23*n*, 31*n*, 42, 51, 53, 221–
22
Measles, reduces incidence of childbed
fever, 206
Mechanical devices, use of in delivery,
14. *See also* Forceps
Medical: procedures as causes of
childbed fever, 73–74, 84; studies at
the University of Vienna, 104–5,
122, 163; theory, 26–28, 47–48;
theory and social role of physician,
7
Medullary cancer, patient with, a source
of decaying organic matter: discussed, 43–44, 93; mentioned, 106,

114, 117, 119, 124, 171, 185, 193, 194. *See also* Cancer of the uterus; Carcinoma

Meningitis, 87, 88

Menstruation, as a cause of childbed fever, 229

Metritis, 191, 226

Metrophlebitis, 152, 191, 231

Metrorrhagia, as a cause of childbed fever, 246

Meyrhofer, Karl, 56n

Miasmata, as causes of childbed fever, 12, 14, 16, 33, 158–59, 182, 199, 200, 208–11 passim, 221, 226, 232, 246, 249. *See also* Effluvia; Nosocomial atmosphere

Michaelis, Gustav Adolph: mentioned, 30n, 51n, 172, 178, 179, 180; quoted, 129, 137, 176–77

Midwives: Hungarian, more enlightened than Virchow, 232–33; practices of Viennese, 81, 126n; student, in Paris, 125

Milk fever, 232

Milk secretion, as a cause of childbed fever, 246

Modesty, offense to, as a cause of childbed fever, 73, 79, 80, 160–61

Mikschik, Eduard, 49, 123–24

Müller, Terézia, 16

Munich: 127; maternity hospital, 232–36

Murphy, Edward William, 21, 35, 175, 175n

Nail brushes, use of in disinfection, 3, 238, 238n

Natural obstetrics, 154. *See also* Boër, Rogers Lucas Johann

Necessary conditions: for childbed fever, 30, 31, 32, 36, 37, 43, 49–53; in disease causation, 28, 38

Nervous fever, a euphemism for women's diseases, 242

Newborn, childbed fever among the:

discussed, 18–19, 45–47, 77–79, 99; mentioned, 38, 40, 49, 80, 86, 88, 100, 117, 206, 229

Nosocomial atmosphere, as a cause of childbed fever, 226, 226n, 230. *See also* Effluvia; Miasmata

Noxious humors, 12

Nuland, Sherwin B., 51n, 52n, 58

Nursing, in relation to childbed fever, 232

Obstetrical clinics. *See* Maternity clinics

Official correspondence, Semmelweis's, regarding unsanitary conditions, 110–13

Operative intervention, as a cause of childbed fever, 247

Osiander, Johann Friedrich: mentioned, 74n, 128; quoted, 125, 153

Overcrowding, as a cause of childbed fever, 17, 69–70, 127, 158, 178–79, 190, 233

Paderborn maternity clinic, 34, 228

Paid maternity ward, in Vienna, 123–24

Paralysis of the lungs, a euphemism for women's diseases, 242

Pasteur, Louis, 55

Pathological anatomy, 26, 29, 118–19, 152, 222, 226; general principles of, 8, 18–19, 77; Semmelweis's argument as a repudiation of, 25, 45–48, 49

Patient with: carious knee, 43–44, 93, 106, 114, 116, 117, 119, 171, 185, 193, 194; gangrenous genitals, 113, 113n, 148–49; medullary cancer, 43–44, 93, 106, 114, 117, 119, 124, 171, 185, 193, 194

Pericarditis, 87, 88, 206

Perineal lacerations, as a source of decaying organic matter, 166

Period of dilation, in relation to onset

Period of dilation (*continued*)
  of childbed fever, 76–77, 86, 98–99, 196, 207
Peritonitis, 87, 88, 226, 230
Pest: maternity clinic, 62, 108–13, 115, 116, 129, 130, 148, 154, 195, 213; mentioned, 56, 106
Petition: Scanzoni's, to investigate childbed fever, 198–200; Semmelweis's, to improve facilities in Pest clinic, 108–10, 118
Peu, Phillipe, 152–53
Phlebitis, 87, 204
Plethora, 15; as a cause of childbed fever, 76, 161, 246
Pleurisy, 87, 88, 206
Pneumonia, 11, 206
Polyp of the uterus, 218–19
Postpartum uterine contractions, in relation to the onset of childbed fever, 231–32
Prague: cases of childbed fever reported in, 134–36, maternity hospital 191–214 passim, 232, 240; mentioned, 175
Predisposing factors, for childbed fever, 34, 79–80, 204, 249. *See also* Childbed fever, cause of
Pregnancy: as a cause of childbed fever, 161, 229; blood mixture characteristic of, 204, 206; fever in, as a cause of childbed fever, 246; occurrence of childbed fever during, 16, 18, 83, 115–16, 117, 204
Premature deliveries, in relation to childbed fever, 40, 82–83, 86, 100–101, 206
Private physicians, lower incidence of childbed fever in practice of, 141
Private ward, in Viennese maternity hospital, 17
Prophylaxis of disease, 27, 28. *See also* Childbed fever, prophylaxis and therapy of; Chlorine washings
Providence, as an explanation for childbed fever, 13, 13n, 160n

Pychogenic hydrophobia, 27n
Puerperal fever. *See* Childbed fever
Puerperal processes, 9n
Purgatives, as a treatment for childbed fever, 14, 129
Putrid fever, as a source of decaying organic matter, 248
Pyemia: among surgeons and anatomists, 19n, 117, 206; in relation to childbed fever, 41, 49, 51n, 105, 117, 168, 181–82, 229, 241; mentioned, 58, 191, 204, 213, 239; Semmelweis's characterization of, 38, 197–98, 229

Rabies. *See* Hydrophobia
Reedal, G., 145
Religious practices, as causes of childbed fever, 71–73
Repercussion, Skoda pioneered, 82n
Resorption, of decaying animal-organic matter. *See* Childbed fever, cause of, decaying animal-organic matter as
Rheumatic fever, 80
Rheumatism, 206
Rigby, Edward, 138
Roberton, John, 144, 146
Rokitansky, Karl: biographical note, 95n; in relation to Semmelweis, 48–49, 51–53, 95, 102; mentioned, 18, 22–25 passim, 54, 95, 105, 128, 170n
Rough treatment by physicians, as a cause of childbed fever, 17, 73, 84, 101, 103
Routh, C. H. G.: mentioned, 21, 32, 34, 35, 42, 115n, 175n; quoted, 30, 174–75

St. Rochus hospital: described, 106–8; mentioned, 56, 112, 117, 129, 130, 154, 212
Salles, a physician reporting on childbed fever in South America, 151
Scandinavian hospitals, incidence of childbed fever in, 243
Scanzoni, Wilhelm Friedrich: men-

tioned, 31, 53, 232, 239; quoted and discussed, 33, 191–214

Scarlet fever compared with childbed fever, 117, 206

Schmidt, Joseph Hermann: mentioned, 34, 230; quoted and discussed, 225–28

Scholz, a physician reporting on childbed fever in Jerusalem, 151

Schwartz, Heinrich Hermann, mentioned, 30, 51n, 137, 179, 180

Scientific theories, nature of, 224

Scotland, occurrence of childbed fever in, 133, 139, 156

Scurvy, reduces incidence of childbed fever, 206

Seasons, influences of, on childbed fever, 15, 40, 67, 122–23, 157, 242. *See also* Climate; Weather

Self-infection: as a cause of childbed fever, 29, 44–45, 114, 116, 118, 119; mentioned, 39, 120, 141, 150, 154, 162, 163, 165, 198, 205, 207, 212, 228, 247; prevention of, 166

Semmelweis, Ignaz: attitude toward women in medicine, 6, 232–33; biographical information about, 16, 21–25, 28–32, 56–58, 61, 63–113 passim, 168, 218–19, 222; Budapest lectures, 36n; contribution to medical theory, 6–8; final illness, 57–58, 170n, 233n; influence on subsequent thought, 53–55; May 15 lecture, 19n, 23, 23n, 31n, 32–35, 42, 51, 53, 210, 221–22; mentioned by critics and supporters, 32, 33, 35, 41, 171–72, 173, 177, 180, 182, 183, 184, 185, 196, 209, 210, 212, 217, 219, 221, 223, 224, 226, 237, 238n; opposition to, 22, 23, 24, 32–36 passim, 41–48, 168–251 passim; open letters, 57; relative priority of, 3, 7, 42–43, 52; sources of his views on childbed fever, 48–53

Semmelweis, József, 16

Sepsis, of the blood, 100

Septic fever, in relation to childbed fever, 189

Sequential cases, of childbed fever, 83, 86, 93, 101

Sexual norms, 5–6

Seyfert, Bernhard, mentioned, 31, 194n, 209, 210

Shame, as a cause of childbed fever, 14, 16

Silberschmidt, H., quoted and discussed, 212–13

Simpson, James Young: biographical note, 174n; his response to Semmelweis, 42; mentioned, 30, 207; quoted and discussed 174–76

Simultaneous illness, as a cause of childbed fever, 229–30

Skoda, Josef: biographical note, 82n; lectures on Semmelweis's discovery, 30–31, 190–91, 217, 219; mentioned, 36n, 82, 95, 146, 170n, 192n, 209, 212, 213, 237; relation to Semmelweis 19n, 21–24, 30–31, 32, 34, 42, 48–53, 115n, 196–97

Sleight, R. P., 145

Smallpox, compared with childbed fever, 117, 147, 150, 206

Social role of physician, and medical theory, 7

Social classes, in relation to incidence of childbed fever, 144, 241–42

Sources of decaying animal-organic matter, 114–15, 136, 185, 194–96, 212–13, 218

Späth, Joseph: biographical note, 135n; mentioned, 25n, 57n, 135, 240, 242

Spontaneous cases of disease, 13n, 241

Sporadic cases of childbed fever, 12, 29, 83, 192n

Stasis, as a cause of childbed fever, 246

Steiner, Joseph, quoted, 214–15

Stethoscope, 82n

Stoltz, Joseph-Alexis, 126–28

Stores, Robert, 144–46

Strasbourg: maternity hospital, 69, 126–29, 156; mentioned, 21

Street births: explained, 80–82, 100–101; mentioned, 40, 86, 196, 206, 242–43

Sufficient conditions for childbed fever, 37, 216

Supine deliveries, 18, 87

Supportive treatment for childbed fever, 15

Surgeons, as victims of childbed fever, 117, 148, 204, 229 *See also* Pyemia, among anatomists and surgeons

Surgical fever, identical with childbed fever, 175–76

Surgical patients, in relation to childbed fever, 106–7, 114, 148, 175–76, 189, 204, 206, 229

Symptomatic characterizations of diseases, 25–28 passim, 39

Synchondrosis, 135

Taban, 16. *See also* Budapest

Telluric influences, as causes of childbed fever, 65

Temkin, Owsei, quoted, 55

Tenon, Jacobus-Rene, quoted, 153

Tetanus, 25

Therapeutic nihilism, 186n

Therapy for childbed fever, 14–15, 15n, 63, 134, 137, 189, 234

Thrombosis, in relation to childbed fever, 230–232, 246

Tilanus, Christian Bernard: mentioned, 30, 34, 36n, 172; quoted, 188–90

Tuberculosis, reduces incidence of childbed fever, 206

Typhoid fever, in relation to childbed fever, 11, 36, 46n, 145, 206, 235, 242

Typhus. *See* Typhoid fever

Uncleanliness of the bowel, as a cause of childbed fever, 24n, 129

University of Pest, 56, 108

University of Vienna, 16, 103

University of Zurich, 56

Uremia, as a cause of childbed fever, 246

Uterine contractions, in relation to childbed fever, 231–32

Vascular engorgement, as a cause of childbed fever, 246

Veit, Aloys Constantin Conrad Gustav, 244

Venice, 87, 88

Ventilation, in relation to childbed fever, 17, 75, 127, 138–39, 158, 162, 165, 179, 244, 247–48

Vienna: described, 80, 80n, 122; mentioned, 23, 24, 58, 80, 80n, 122, 152, 156, 170n, 174; University of, 16, 103

Viennese: Academy of Science, 190, 217, 226; practices of, midwives, 81, 126n

—foundling home: admission to, 4, 80–81; childbed fever at, 100, mentioned, 77

—maternity hospital, specifically mentioned, 16, 17, 63, 94, 102, 140, 142–43, 154, 166, 193, 226, 243, 244. *See also* Maternity clinics, first and second, in Vienna

—medical school, 48, 88, 152, 170n. *See also* Medical, studies at the University of Vienna

Virchow, Rudolf: mentioned, 6; quoted and discussed, 228–33, 244

Waldeyer, Wilhelm, mentioned, 56n

Wagensteen, Owen H. and Sarah D., cited, 55

Washing, with soap and water insufficient, 88, 93, 173, 237

Weather, in relation to childbed fever, 188, 189, 208, 229–30 *See also* Climate; Seasons

Webster, John, mentioned, 175

Weidenhoffer, Maria, mentioned, 56, 57

Weiger, Friedrich: biographical note,

126n; discussed, 29n, 36n; mentioned, 21, 51n; quoted, 126
Widgen, Mrs., a British midwife, 138
Winter, in relation to onset of childbed fever, 230, 232. *See also* Seasons
Wittelshofer, Leopold, 24n
Women's diseases, 5

Würzburg: maternity hospital, 165–66; mentioned, 31, 169

Zipfl, Franz: discussed, 221–23, 240; mentioned, 105, 209–10
Zymotic illnesses, 248–49

JACKET DESIGNED BY FRANK WILLIAMS
COMPOSED BY GRAPHIC COMPOSITION, INC.
ATHENS, GEORGIA
MANUFACTURED BY MALLOY LITHOGRAPHING, INC.
ANN ARBOR, MICHIGAN

Library of Congress Cataloging in Publication Data
Semmelweis, Ignác Fülöp, 1818–1865.
The etiology, concept, and prophylaxis of
childbed fever.
(Wisconsin publications in the history of science
and medicine ; no. 2)
Translation of: Die Aetiologie, der Begriff und
die Prophylaxis des Kindbettfiebers.
Includes bibliographical references and index.
1. Puerperal septicemia. 2. Asepsis and antisepsis.
I. Carter, K. Codell (Kay Codell), 1939–
II. Title. III. Series. [DNLM: 1. Puerperal infection
—Etiology. 2. Septicemia—Prevention and control. W1
WI805 no. 2 / WQ S472a]
RG811.S4313 1983   618.7′4   83–47758
ISBN 0-299-09360-3
ISBN 0-299-09364-6 (pbk.)